A PATIENT'S GUIDE TO MEDICAL AESTHETICS

Dr Harry Singh
BChD (Leeds), MFGDP (UK)

All rights reserved. © Dr Harry Singh 2019

No part of this document may be reproduced, sold, stored in or introduced into a retrieval system, or transmitted, in any form or by any means (electronic, mechanical, photocopying, recording or otherwise), without the prior permission of the copyright owner.

First printing: 2019

ISBN-13: 9781070639857

British Cataloguing Publication Data:
A catalogue record of this book is available from The British Library.

Contents

Disclaimer 5

Introduction 7

Chapter 1: Trends in non-surgical aesthetic treatments
.... 8

    1.1 Statistics 9

    1.2 Most popular treatments............................ 11

    1.3 Top reasons why people seek treatments 13

    1.4 Benefits of treatments 14

    1.5 Regulation 22

    1.6 Things you should check before having an aesthetic treatment 28

    1.7 Aesthetics patient charter............................ 30

    1.8 Myths about treatments............................... 32

Chapter 2: Attractiveness...................................... 34

    2.1 Attractiveness... 35

    2.2 Gender differences 36

    2.3 Cultural differences 37

Chapter 3: Ageing... 38

    3.1 Skin 39

    3.2 Fat 45

    3.3 Bone.. 46

    3.4 Decade by decade 47

Chapter 4: Injectables 50

    4.1 Botox 51

    4.2 Dermal fillers 79

Chapter 5: Skin 103

    5.1 Good skin 104

    5.2 Sun Damage 108

    5.3 Myths about moisturisers 112

    5.4 Cosmeceuticals 116

    5.5 Sunekos 121

    5.6 Threads 124

Chapter 6: Body 130

    6.1 Fat dissolving 131

    6.2. Cellulite 136

    6.3. IV vitamins 139

About the Author 142

References 146

Disclaimer

Please seek independent medical advice and thoroughly research the benefits and risks associated before embarking on any procedure. This book is designed as a source of information and is not intended to give any specific advice.

Introduction

With the ever-increasing exposure to medical aesthetics and the increase in popularity in these procedures, there seems to be a lot of misinformation and confusion.

I felt a non-biased guide to the benefits, risks, costs, comfort levels and duration of results was needed to educate you, the consumer.

This book is for anyone who:

- is confused as to where to start
- is unsure whether to take the plunge
- wants a clear pathway of what is available to them

This book is divided into the following categories:

Trends
Attractiveness
Ageing process
Injectables
Skin
Body

For more information and to book a free consultation please visit www.aesthetics-dentistry.com

Chapter 1: Trends in non-surgical aesthetic treatments

1.1 Statistics

1.2 Most popular treatments

1.3 Top reasons why people seek treatments

1.4 Benefits of treatments

1.5 Regulation

1.6 Things you should check before getting an aesthetic treatment

1.7 Aesthetics patient charter

1.8 Myths about treatments

1.1 Statistics

In 2013, the Department of Health predicted that the value of the cosmetic surgery industry in the UK would rise from £2.3bn in 2010 to £3.6bn in 2015. This is certainly something that many dentists are becoming more interested in offering their patients, since they are ideally placed, once appropriately trained, to deliver non-surgical facial aesthetics complementary to dental treatment.

The trend today is away from traditional cosmetic surgery and towards less expensive, minimally invasive procedures.[1] The use of cosmetic procedures to reduce the signs of ageing has increased dramatically over the past 10 years. You may be wondering why a dentist would be working in non-surgical facial aesthetics. The truth is that dentists are actually ideally placed to perform such treatments, since we have undergone five years of undergraduate education focusing just on the face, never mind the postgraduate training that inevitably follows!

A large part of what we learn involves not just teeth but also the anatomical structures allied to the mouth, as well as providing oral treatment that is in proportion with the patient's face, We are also experts at administering pain-free injections.

We dentists, just like any other healthcare professional

that patients see on a regular basis, are in the fortunate position of being able to build rapport and therefore trust. Who better then to deliver non-surgical facial aesthetic treatments?

1.2 Most popular treatments

Much like tattoos and piercings, aesthetic procedures are becoming commonplace in society. Whether it's celebrities we see on TV or just regular people in the street, there are a host of procedures that people from all walks of life are undertaking in order to increase their confidence and make them feel better about themselves.

Botox – we've all heard of Botox, but some people may be unsure what it actually is. Botulinum Toxin injections are medical treatments that relax facial muscles and help fight the signs of ageing. By making lines and wrinkles less obvious, Botox injections can make you look younger and healthier without the need for surgery.

Lip fillers – arguably one of the biggest cosmetic trends in the world, lip fillers have had a meteoric rise in popularity over the past few years due to celebrities such as Kylie Jenner. Fillers can alter the shape of the lips and give them more volume. As we get older, our lips deplete and become thinner; lip enhancement procedures can help reverse these symptoms.

Jawline fillers – as you grow older, you may notice your jawline has lost its definition and is not as tight or shapely as it was previously. Thankfully, the rise in modern medical procedures means you can have jawline fillers injected in order to give your jaw more definition and give your face that youthful appearance we're all chasing.

Cheek fillers – sagging skin is a part of life that affects us all, but thankfully, we can now fight ageing skin on our face. Voluminous cheeks give the face a much more youthful appearance and cheek fillers can help give your cheeks volume and eradicate the obvious signs of ageing.

Facial peels – these are liquids that are brushed onto the skin to remove dead skin cells and promote the growth of new cells. The procedure can reduce ageing spots and even out skin tone, making skin appear youthful and healthy.

1.3 Top reasons why people seek treatments

- To look good on social media/Facebook
- To improve their social status
- To improve their professional/work image
- To follow a fashionable trend
- To feel better about themselves
- To compete with other women/men of similar or younger ages
- To be more attractive to their partners

1.4 Benefits of treatments

While ageing is just a fact of life that we have to contend with, there are certain procedures that can battle the signs of ageing and help us keep our youthful appearance for longer. The benefits of aesthetics don't stop there – there are many other benefits to undergoing aesthetic procedures, with some being more publicised than others.

Established in 2014 and created by the award-winning Dr Harry Singh, The Botulinum Toxin Club is the UK's leading facial aesthetics training workshop for dentists, doctors, medics, specialists and nurses. Together, they share five surprising benefits of aesthetics with their patients – and now with you.

Improved self-confidence – aesthetic procedures such as Botox and lip fillers help us look younger, smoother and healthier, which can lead to an increase in self-confidence. Not only will you feel more confident in yourself, but this will also radiate through you and change the way other people view and engage with you.

It improves your mood – not only will your increased self-confidence improve your mood, but facial expressions can also send certain feedback to the brain and result in the changing of your mood. Emotions such as fear, sadness or anger can result in the contraction of muscles in the forehead that cause frown lines. By blocking these frowning muscles with Botox, you may also improve your mood.

You'll receive more compliments – we all like to be complimented from time to time, but you're unlikely to receive positive feedback on your eye-wrinkles and thin lips. Procedures such as Botox and lip fillers will make you look younger and more radiant, leading to more compliments and attention.

It's not just for the ladies – aesthetic procedures such as facial fillers are commonly associated with women, but they can also greatly benefit men. Male aesthetic procedures are becoming increasingly popular, with men claiming the procedures help them get ahead at work, even resulting in an increase in sales.

It makes you more health-conscious – aesthetic procedures often lead to an increased interest in our appearance, which leads to more health-conscious decisions. Seeing yourself looking young may be the push you need to start pursuing a more active and healthier lifestyle in general.

Can our moods be affected by Botulinum Toxin?

Did the chicken or egg come first?

Does our mood reflect our facial expressions - or do our facial expressions reflect our mood?

We always assumed that our emotions directed our facial expressions, but studies have suggested it is in fact our facial expressions that determine our emotions.[2]

You cannot feel depressed if you are smiling and being expressive with your face. To feel depressed, you need to have little expression on your face, look sad, look down and curl up your body. Whenever my children are upset or start crying, the first thing I do is to get them to open their body up and look towards to the sky. Then I crack a joke to get them to smile, and it works every time. Researchers also understood the above strategy and started asking themselves whether we could change a person's mood and help decrease depression if we prevented a negative facial expression, such as frowning.

William James, an American philosopher, postulated in 1890 that the common sense of viewing emotions is wrong. He went on to say that if our body is unable to express an emotion, that emotion ceases to exist. For example, we cannot experience fear without a faster heartbeat, more shallow breathing, trembling lips, going weak at the knees, goosebumps, etc.

Our facial expressions have evolved over millions of years. In 1872, Charles Darwin wrote: "A man may be absorbed in the deepest thought, and his brow will remain smooth until he encounters some obstacle in his train of reasoning, or is interrupted by some disturbance, and then a frown passes like a shadow over his brow."[3]

We can all tell if someone is angry by their negative facial expression, such as frowning. We know the opposite to the negative frown is the positive smile.

> *"A smile cures the wounding of a frown."*
> *Shakespeare*

There are different types of smiles but a truly genuine smile has been classified as the 'Duchenne smile'. In 1860, Duchenne, a French anatomist, observed the 'smile of joy', where the orbicularis oculi is activated and contracts to produce crow's feet. This is in stark contrast to the 'Mona Lisa smile', where the eyes are not involved at all. Very few people can fake a genuine smile. Smiling is good for us. Smiling creates positive emotions and thus leads to a reduction in stress-related hormones.

A third type of smile is known as Hawthorne's 'sad smile'. When you are experiencing a sad/depressing event – let's say a funeral – and you see a relative who is struggling to cope with the circumstances, this is the small smile you may give them to indicate we are in this together and we will be ok.

Let's go back and look at the negative facial expression of frowning. There are different types of frowns (sad versus angry) depending on which muscles are recruited, and each one has a different meaning. If the inner part of your eyebrows points upwards whilst frowning, you will look sad. If, however, the eyebrows are drawn together and down whilst frowning, you will look angry.

Frowning occurs through the contraction of the glabellar muscles, of which there are two major ones – the corrugator supercilii and the procerus. It is the corrugator supercilii that contributes more to the frown. Translated from Latin, corrugator supercilii literally means 'the wrinkler above the eye' and the contraction of this muscle draws the eyebrows together to create the frown. We all know the appearance of a frown will show others exactly what you are feeling, but let's take it a step further: the actual process of frowning will tell *you* what you are feeling and this creates a state in your conscious mind which will influence your decisions and your results.

Recent research has put flesh on the bones of these musings. Neurobiologists such as Antonio Damasio of the University of Southern California have demonstrated that emotions begin with actions – rapidly increased heart rate, for example – and end with the perception of those actions – the sensation of fear or anger. Damasio calls this the 'body loop': the brain learns of the body's response to change via chemical and electric signals conveyed by the bloodstream and nervous system. Thus, feeling follows behaviour; the mind follows the body.

I break this down using the acronym T.E.A.R.

Everything starts with Thoughts. Thoughts spark off certain Emotions, which lead us into Action, which eventually determines our Results. We can see that our initial thoughts determine the results we achieve in life.

If we are postulating that it's your facial expressions that determine your emotions and mood at any given time, where can we seek evidence for this? Hollywood. Actors have to take up various roles and associated moods on a regular basis. As far back as the 18th century, a German dramatist Gotthold Ephraim suggested that, "the actor properly imitates all the external signs… and all the bodily… expressions of a particular (inner) state," and therefore they will recreate internally the exact same emotions, thoughts and feelings of the acted part. This began the research into 'facial feedback'.

Charles Ball, in Essays on the Anatomy and Philosophy of Expression, wrote, "By the actions and expressions of the body betraying the passions of the heart we may be startled and forewarned, as it were, by the reflection of ourselves, and at the same time learn to control our passions by restraining the expression of them."

Charles Darwin then described "the intimate relation which exists between almost all the emotions and their outward manifestation and partly from the direct influence of exertion on the heart, and consequently on the brain."

In 1890, Harvard psychologist William James in his work 'Principles of Psychology' suggested that our muscles contribute to our emotions and that changes in the muscles are occurring all the time to suit the emotions of the moment, even if we are consciously unaware of them.

More recent studies have shown a correlation between the intensity of the smile and the internal emotion it produces.

We all want to be happier and reduce the amount of stress we experience. How can we do this?

One simple way is to smile more and have more positive thoughts. This will lift your mood and limit the production of any negative facial expressions.

What about the use of Botulinum Toxin? Eric Finzi carried out Botulinum Toxin treatments on patients who were depressed but showed no visible frowns. On review, he noticed that these patients felt a marked improvement in their emotional state. He postulates that the contraction of these frown muscles sends negative emotional signals to the brain; the brain measures the strength of the frown muscle contraction and weighs it against the strength of the smile and thus decides which emotion to produce.

My patients come in for a number of reasons, some cosmetic and some to improve their confidence. I would say it probably does put you in a better mood if you feel better about the way you look. It's like doing your hair, your teeth, whatever else.

It is not what happens to you that is important; it is what you feel and do about what has happened to you.

1.5 Regulation

Currently, there is no regulatory body or any formal process of regulation regarding the administration of non-surgical facial aesthetics. There is no legal requirement to register with any specific non-surgical body, though there are a number of bodies that you can join voluntarily, such as Save Face and JCCP. I expect in the near future compulsory registration to a body, whichever one that may be, will come into effect to help maintain high standards in the delivery of non-surgical aesthetics.

Whilst we are awaiting formal regulation, please only seek treatments from medical professionals who are regulated by their own medical regulatory body.

A bit of history: as a result of the PIP implant scandal, Sir Bruce Keogh was asked by the Department of Health to investigate the cosmetic interventions industry. He was asked to look at:

- Standards for cosmetic surgery practice and training;

- Fillers as a POM (prescription only medicine);

- Registration;

- Accreditation;

- Record of consent;

- Advertising restrictions;

- Professional indemnity cover.

The Keogh report was produced in April 2013 and the government responded to it in February 2014. Work was then started to create documentation and, where necessary, legislation to implement a number of the key recommendations, which included:

- A register of everyone who performs surgical or non-surgical cosmetic interventions;

- Classifying dermal fillers as a prescription only medical device;

- Ensuring all practitioners are properly qualified for all the procedures they offer;

- All non-surgical procedures to be performed under the responsibility of a clinical professional who has gained the accredited qualification to prescribe, administer and supervise aesthetic procedures;

- A ban on special financial offers for surgery;

- An advertising code of conduct with mandatory compliance for practitioners;

- Compulsory professional indemnity in case things go wrong;

- An ombudsman to oversee all private healthcare, including cosmetic procedures, to help those who have been treated poorly.

In 2015, Health Education England (HEE) was commissioned by the Department of Health to develop guidance reports outlining the qualification requirements for the delivery of a number of non-surgical cosmetic interventions and hair restoration surgical procedures with the aim of improving and standardising the training available to practitioners.

The qualification requirements include areas of study that were highlighted as key requirements in the Keogh review, such as training on obtaining informed consent, information governance and record keeping, and ensuring that practitioners have a clear understanding of the requirement to operate from safe premises, with patient safety training in topics such as infection control, treatment room safety and adverse incident reporting. They also address recommendations for training in physiology, anatomy, infection control, treatment of anaphylaxis and an understanding of existing medical conditions so that practitioners are aware of all the possible risks and complications of the procedures and are able to recognise and treat complications.

The qualification requirements correspond with different levels of learning which reflect the complexity and risk level of different procedures and the corresponding knowledge and skills requirements identified to ensure patient/client safety and high standards of care. The levels go from Level 4 to Level 7 and those with a dental, medical or nursing degree will automatically be at Level 6.

Ofqual are currently determining what is required to make a practitioner Level 7 competent. The main addition to current training pathways is mentoring. There will be a number of cases that the practitioner will need to observe and a number of cases where a trainer will observe the practitioner at work.

Dr Harry Singh is one of only a few practitioners nationwide who has successfully passed and is qualified to offer this Level 7 training to other medical practitioners.

The Joint Council for Cosmetic Practitioners (JCCP) was set up recently to group together dentists, doctors and medical nurses in a united front to discuss the two guidance reports produced by the HEE. The JCCP wants to take the lead role in terms of requirements for training and ongoing standards for delivering non-surgical aesthetics rather than be dictated to by the HEE. These discussions are ongoing, so watch this space!

Advertising

There are three bodies that are responsible for promoting prescription only medicines (POM) such as Botox®.

www.asa.org.uk: Advertising Standards Authority (ASA) – ASA looks at how practitioners describe and promote what they offer.

www.cap.org.uk: Committee of Advertising Practice (CAP) – CAP has produced a document on 'Marketing of Cosmetic Interventions'.

www.mhra.gov.uk: Medicines and Healthcare Products (MHRA) – Regulatory agency MHRA deals with the ordering, storage and dispensing of POMs.

The future will reinforce and introduce new methods to protect the public and this has already started with surgical procedures, with the introduction of the cooling off period. I foresee this crossing over to non-surgical aesthetics soon.

The GMC has already taken the initiative and produced guidance for doctors who offer cosmetic interventions, which can be found at

http://www.gmc-uk.org/guidance/ethical_guidance/28687.asp

In summary, this guidance looks at advertising responsibly, giving patients time for reflection, not delegating the consent process, having detailed notes and monitoring quality and outcomes.

What about treatment-wise and services-wise? We have already progressed from line chasing (a few Botox® jabs) to a full face approach combining anti-wrinkle treatments with dermal fillers and skin treatments to offer a full holistic approach. I feel we will build on the whole face/body approach as new technology and services come to the forefront, like whole body nutrition procedures such as vitamin infusions, and possibly have a one stop shop for all your non-surgical aesthetics, whether it be for your face or body.

1.6 Things you should check before having an aesthetic treatment

With more people than ever before having aesthetic procedures, it's become increasingly common to hear of untrained professionals performing these complex procedures, resulting in horrific results that often go viral online. For this reason, you need to make sure you research the clinic before going for a procedure.

According to the Botulinum Toxin Club, here are five things you should check before booking an aesthetic treatment:

Are they professional? – before you have any procedures, make sure you check whether the person carrying it out is a professional. Sadly, due to the rising popularity in aesthetic procedures, con artists and scammers are seeing an opportunity to make money out of other people's misery. Make sure the practitioner you choose is a medical professional and not a chancer.

Check for qualifications – one way to make sure someone is a professional is to check the qualifications they have and whether they have indemnity insurance. Ask to see evidence that they are a registered medical professional and have attended industry-recognised workshops to learn the required skills to carry out the procedure. If they can't provide evidence, do not use their services.

Read testimonials – if your doctor is trustworthy and professional, they should have testimonials online from clients who have used their services in the past. Check for reviews on Google, Facebook and other online directories to ensure they can give you the experience you require. If there are no reviews online, warning bells should begin to ring.

Look at the environment – Botox and fillers are medical procedures, so they need to be undertaken in a clean, clinical environment. If you are unsure about the cleanliness of the environment, don't run the risk and look for a new, cleaner clinic instead.

Is there an option for a cooling off period? – given that aesthetics procedures are fairly serious procedures carried out by medical professionals, there needs to be an option for a cooling off period, allowing you to never feel rushed into committing to the procedure. If your doctor rushes you, that shows an unprofessional side to them and it may be best to avoid using their services.

1.7 Aesthetics patient charter

This is an example of our own patient charter which we follow religiously. Make sure any clinic you are considering using has a similarly robust charter in place.

Our aim is total patient satisfaction. To achieve this aim, we:

Provide skin rejuvenation treatments and advice to high standards

Maintain confidentiality of all patients

Use techniques and materials for which we have had specific training

Provide a continuum of care to include referrals to other professional colleagues where appropriate

Maintain infection control to the highest standards by following the latest professional guidelines

Seek improvement in patient comfort for all aesthetic medical treatments through local anaesthesia

Maintain full and confidential treatment records including before and after treatment photographs

Ensure that patients fully understand proposed treatments and have the opportunity to give informed written consent

Provide suitable guidance and aftercare following treatment

Stay abreast of the latest facial aesthetic techniques through regular training, the reading of professional literature and information provided by professional bodies

Audit our clinical results and review patient satisfaction on a regular basis

1.8 Myths about treatments

With the rise in popularity of aesthetic procedures, we're now seeing more botch jobs and awful results appear online. While there are certain dangers that come with these treatments, if they are carried out correctly, they can enhance your confidence and give you a new lease of life. But, despite the positive impact of aesthetic procedures, there are still quite a few myths surrounding them.

Here are five of the most common myths about aesthetic procedures.

The 'frozen look' – when people hear the word 'Botox,' they often associate it with a frozen face that shows little to no expression. But, while Botox does iron out facial creases and wrinkles, it doesn't have to lead to a completely 'frozen' look. Botox injections are fully controlled, meaning you can choose the dosage you receive.

It's permanent – many people believe that Botox is permanent, meaning if you do end up with the frozen look, you'll be stuck like that forever. The truth is, however, Botox does not last forever and requires regular updates and top-ups. If you are unhappy with your results, rest easy in the fact that it won't last forever.

It's not reversible – while some fillers and aesthetic

treatments are irreversible, certain lip fillers can be reversed. Hyaluronic acid-based fillers, such as the Juvéderm that Kylie Jenner famously used, are reversible. Make sure you check which medicines are being used and whether they can be reversed.

It's expensive – aesthetic procedures used to be associated with the rich and famous, but this is no longer the case. The majority of procedures are now affordable and available for purchase by the general public, with many costing only a few hundred pounds.

Anyone can do it – whatever you do, never believe that anyone can perform aesthetic procedures. While your local salon may claim they can perform aesthetic treatments, unless they have a qualified professional who has undergone extensive training, it's not worth running the risk. Only recognised and trusted professionals should carry out these treatments.

Chapter 2: Attractiveness

2.1 Attractiveness

2.2 Gender differences

2.3 Cultural differences

2.1 Attractiveness

What makes an attractive face – and is there some magic formula or proportion that, if adhered to, we would all find attractive?

Nature always followed the Golden Ratio, which is denoted by the Greek symbol 'phi' and relates to the numerical value of 1.618.

Therefore, it would make sense that following this ratio would create an attractive face. But this is not always the case. Study the faces of attractive celebrities – take Angelina Jolie, for example: you will no doubt see her face does not follow the Golden Ratio at all!

Further research shows that it is not actually the Golden Ratio that determines whether a face is likely to be perceived as more or less attractive; rather, it's the symmetry between both sides of the face. The more symmetrical the face, the more attractive you will be deemed to be.

2.2 Gender differences

In a blog published by The Association for Psychological Science, titled 'Beauty is in the Mind of the Beholder', they discuss the role of attractiveness in our lives and the decisions we make.

An attractive man, in the eyes of female experimental participants, is generally one with relatively prominent cheekbones and eyebrow ridges and a relatively long lower face. Likewise, prominent cheekbones, large eyes, small nose, a taller forehead, smooth skin, and an overall young or even childlike appearance add to women's allure in the eyes of male raters.

2.3 Cultural differences

Just as fashion and food trends are different in different parts of the world, it's no surprise that what determines attractiveness in different parts of the world significantly varies too.

In an e-book produced by Galderma, 'The Changing Face of Aesthetic Treatments', the author highlights cultural differences in the ageing process, such as fewer wrinkles appearing in darker skin because of the thickness of the skin.

When it comes to facial aesthetics, different cultures will have different requirements because of the genetic nature of their background, such as:

- Asian skin will have a genetic predisposition to dark circles around the eyes.

- Darker skinned people will have naturally fuller lips.

- Oriental females may have more masculine features, such as a square jaw appearance and smaller eyes.

In conclusion, when it comes to facial aesthetics it's important that every face is approached as unique.

Chapter 3: Ageing

3.1 Skin

3.2 Fat

3.3 Bone

3.4 Decade by decade

3.1 Skin

The facial ageing process begins with surface and subsurface structural changes in multiple facial tissue layers, including skin, fat, muscle and bone.

Facial tissue layers age interdependently, contributing to the overall facial appearance.

As we get older, the structure of our skin changes and we experience:

- thinning of the skin
- loss of collagen
- loss of elastin
- decreased hyaluronic acid production

These changes can be evidenced in our skin in the following ways:

- Loss of elasticity
- Increased dryness

As time passes our skin succumbs to a perfectly natural ageing process. The effects of pollution, stress, fatigue and toxins leave their mark and the skin loses its suppleness and elasticity. Nothing reflects our age more than the state of our skin.

The key to growing old gracefully is through good living and awareness of your environment. While many of the changes that come with skin ageing can't be avoided, some can definitely be minimised. First, it helps to have a basic understanding of what happens to the skin as it goes through the ageing process.

The skin ages in two key ways: intrinsic and extrinsic.

Intrinsic ageing is genetically predetermined – you can't avoid it. Eventually the skin gets thinner, drier and less elastic. This happens because we produce less collagen over time. The drop in collagen production also causes skin to sag and become less able to bounce back with weight loss or gain.

The reason skin gets dryer and thinner over time is because the dermis (deep layer of the skin) loses its ability to hold or attract water. On top of this, age causes a marked decrease in the sweat glands and the oil-producing sebaceous glands. Oils, water and sweat are the elements of moist, plump skin.

Although the onset of these changes varies from person to person, skin ageing usually first becomes apparent in our 30s.

Extrinsic ageing is directly related to exposure to toxins and environmental elements. As you probably know, the sun is one of the biggest culprits behind extrinsic ageing. It basically intensifies the intrinsic ageing process, causing us to look older than our true age. Sun-related ageing, called 'photo ageing', causes fine lines, wrinkles, age spots (due to pigment changes), enlarged pores, broken capillaries and rough, uneven skin tone and texture.

Our lifestyle is another factor in extrinsic ageing. For example, cigarette smoking not only speeds up the breakdown of collagen and elastin, it causes the formation of skin-killing free radicals (chemically active atoms). Further, it makes it harder for the skin to repair itself.

Poor eating habits also have an effect. A colourful, well-balanced diet is rich in the antioxidants and anti-inflammatories vital for a healthy complexion.

From acne to sensitivity, if your skin is inflamed it won't function properly. An inflamed skin is an unbalanced skin. Inflammation can be caused by lots of trigger factors:

- Stress
- Lack of sleep
- Poor diet
- Dehydration
- Incorrect products

- Over-stimulation
- Sun damage
- Pollution
- Hormones

Keep your skin clean, protected and hydrated and you are on the right path. But make sure you always check the ingredients before buying a product. So many cheap cosmetics bulk up their products with irritating ingredients that can cause all sorts of skin problems and take a while to correct.

Ingredients to avoid include mineral oil, talc, dyes, glycolic acid, benzoyl peroxide and petroleum. These are all common triggers for skin problems. Speak to a skin care consultant if you are suffering with redness, breakouts, sensitivity, heat, dry or cracked skin.

Every moment of exposure to daylight adds up like money in the bank – the problem is the pay off known as sun damage (also known as photo damage). Sun damage shows on skin in the form of wrinkles and hyper pigmentation and can lead to a repressed immune system and the potential for skin cancer.

Even if exposure is limited to brief outdoor lunches or a 20-minute walk, cumulative exposure is enough to cause the signs of skin ageing. The first line of defence against sun damage is daily use of SPF. Even on cloudy or overcast days, UV light can strike skin and cause damage, so simply wearing sunscreen on sunny days isn't enough.

Fortunately, more sophisticated sunscreen formulations with skin health benefits (think less chalky, less greasy) have made SPF a convenient addition to our morning routine. Speak with your professional skin therapist about SPF moisturisers that can be worn comfortably under make-up, or alone to deliver defence against skin ageing UV light.

Exfoliation delivers a tighter, firmer, smoother look and feel to skin and as a result, many people fall into the trap of over-exfoliation: an over-zealous approach that can actually reduce skin's vitality and make it more susceptible to damage from UV light.

Over-exfoliation triggers the inflammatory response, leading to a compromised lipid barrier that won't function properly, a sensitised skin condition, and accelerated premature ageing.

Tell-tale signs of over-exfoliated skin include:

- noticeable dehydration
- patchy areas of dryness
- skin tautness

- redness and itchiness
- increased sensitivity
- inflammatory acne and irritation

If you're showing signs of over-exfoliation, speak with a professional skin therapist, who will most likely prescribe a calming cleanser and toner, and a protective moisturiser to start the recovery process. Sun protection is a must: wear a sunscreen with physical UV blockers titanium dioxide or zinc oxide that won't irritate the skin. After skin recovery, begin exfoliating with a gentle exfoliant designed for daily use. If you desire a more intense level of exfoliation, look to non-abrasive exfoliants containing chemicals like salicylic or lactic acid. Pair a gentler regimen with professional exfoliation treatments from your professional skin therapist to enjoy smoother skin without the undesirable side effects.

Hyper-pigmented conditions occur when the skin produces more melanin than normal, sparking discolouration.

3.2 Fat

When we are younger (in fact, right back to when we were babies), we have large volumes of fat that act as a cushioning layer. As we age, we experience both a decreased volume of fat and the downward displacement of the fat pads underneath the skin.

We have two specific types of fat pad: superficial fat pads, which act as a 'cushion' from external trauma to our skin; and deep fat pads, which shape and mould our face.

As mentioned above, these fat pads begin to descend and deflate and change the structure of our face.

The area most affected by this fat loss as we age is the mid face area, notably the cheeks.

The other area affected dramatically is the jowl area. As the fat pads begin to descend and gravity takes hold, fat begins to accumulate in the jowl area.

3.3 Bone

The bone is the last layer of the face. As we age, there are certain areas of the skull that will gradually start to break down, known in medical terms as 'resorbing'. As the bone shrinks, the layers above the bone, such as the fat and skin layers, will lose support and start sinking inwards.

Certain areas of the face will experience more bone loss than others, such as under the eyes, cheek bones, nose, upper jaw and lower jaw. However, it is interesting to note that as we age the eye socket becomes longer and wider!

3.4 Decade by decade

When it comes to health and the rate of ageing, we used to think that our choices were limited – it's in the genes. Today, however, the ageing process no longer mirrors that of our parents and grandparents.

With modern scientific modalities and recent advancements in medical aesthetics, there often exists a vast difference between a person's chronological age and biological age. It can be hard to distinguish a woman in her twenties from a woman in her forties. Unfortunately, the hands of time swing both ways; we may be 45 chronologically, but biologically, our cells may make us appear 55.

Approximately 36 percent of ageing is due to factors beyond our control – our genes and heritage – but the rest is up to us.

So, what's the secret to achieving beauty at any age?

Good health, quality of life and, of course, great skin care.

In your 20s

Prevention is crucial during this phase of your life. If you didn't have good habits in your teens, now is the time to start. Sunscreen should be a part of your daily skin care regimen, applied in the form of an SPF moisturiser, in order to prevent premature ageing. The body and skin show little change in our twenties, but external factors such as sun exposure, alcohol consumption, poor dietary habits and smoking can have adverse effects on skin down the road. If you prevent damage and protect your skin while in your twenties, your complexion will thank you for decades to come.

In your 30s

Between career moves, busy lifestyles and starting a family, our thirties can bring on a variety of different stressors. Many women at this age are plagued by adult acne and inflammatory skin conditions due to hormonal fluctuations and work-related tension. More evidence of internal change begins to surface as age spots, crow's feet and fine lines appear around the eyes and mouth, but signs of ageing can be curtailed with professional correctives. Undergoing a series of non-wounding peels in conjunction with an at-home treatment regimen of resurfacing products can dramatically reduce the look of blemishes, wrinkles and sun spots, helping you to hold onto your youth.

In your 40s

As we enter our forties, noticeable differences occur as skin begins to lose elasticity. There may be slight sagging around the neck area, and lines that were only visible when you smiled or laughed in your thirties may now be etched into your complexion. Because skin cells take longer to migrate to the surface, encouraging cellular turnover and stimulating collagen production is central to promoting healthier, more youthful-looking skin. Incorporating antioxidants into both your diet and skin care routine will assist in preventing further free radical-induced damage. Look for cleansers, exfoliants and serums infused with vitamins A, C and E and load up on fruits, green vegetables, seeds and nuts.

Over 50

After fifty, the skin's abilities to retain moisture and heal properly are significantly weakened as the body experiences internal changes. Hormonal oscillation and diminished natural reserves in mature and menopausal skin can cause the complexion to appear dry or flaky. Skin care treatments containing essential vitamins, emollients and hormonal regulators are believed to play a role in skin immunity and hydration – they will aid in replenishing the skin's lipid barrier to repair tone and texture, and firm up sagging skin (now found around the forehead, mouth and eyes) to rebuild definition.

Chapter 4: Injectables

4.1 Botox

    Intro
    What is it?
    How does it work?
    What it won't do for you
    Procedure
    Bunny lines
    Smoker's lines
    Sad face
    Gummy smile
    Chin
    Neck
    Bruxism
    Hyperhidrosis
    Celebs

4.2 Dermal Fillers

    Intro
    Nasolabials
    Marionette lines
    Lips
    Cheeks
    Jawline
    Chin
    Temples

4.1 Botox

Introduction

Over the years Botox has increased in popularity in many parts of the United Kingdom. Botox today is seen as an effective and affordable non-surgical anti-ageing cosmetic treatment which can be administered during your lunch hour.

Recent reports have suggested that despite the financial downturn, there has been a 15% increase in the number of adults having facial aesthetic treatments, including Botox. This increase signifies that over one million treatments have been carried out.

Nineteen million men and women in the United Kingdom have undergone some form of anti-ageing treatment since this form of non-surgical anti-ageing procedure became available. A high proportion of these have regular Botox Treatments. Botox is today considered a part of an individual's cosmetic routine.

Botox is considered a safe and highly effective treatment to smooth out fine lines, wrinkles, and frown lines on the face. Botox can also be used for other medical conditions such as bladder control and eye movements.

Botox treatments are often known as the classic 'Lunch Break' treatment. The simplicity of a Botox treatment is appealing, taking around 20 minutes or less to administer. The discomfort and side effects are minimal, meaning you can resume normal activity quickly. Initially, there will be a small amount of swelling and redness around the injected area; this will subside after 10 minutes. Results from the Botox injection will be visible within three to four hours of the treatment taking place. The full effect will take up to 10 days.

If you choose to have any form of Botox treatment, choose a quality practice with a practitioner who is qualified and certified to carry out the procedure and has many years of experience. Most practices will offer a free review and top-up injections if required, two to four weeks after the treatment. Thereafter, treatment is expected to last between three to five months.

What is Botox?

Botox is a naturally occurring protein produced by the bacterium Clostridium Botulinum. In a purified form – as is the case with many drugs/medications, such as Penicillin – Botulinum toxin is a very safe, effective treatment not only used in cosmetic clinics, but also for a number of medical conditions, including migraine and excessive sweating.

All botulinum toxins are prescription only medicines (POM) and can only be prescribed by doctors, dentists and nurses with the prescribing qualification, following a face to face assessment and consultation with the qualified prescriber.

Botox® is a licensed brand of Botulinum toxin A. Other licensed brands include Azzalure®, Dysport®, Xeomin® and Bocouture®.

How does Botox work?

The toxin blocks the transition of chemical messages from the nerve to the muscle so the muscle stays in a resting state for a period of 8 to 12 weeks on average.

This may be only a partial reduction in movement, allowing some remaining movement, or a full block, in which case there is very little remaining muscular movement in the area – this very much depends on the location and amount administered. Treatment may be tailored to suit your individual requirements. Your expected treatment outcomes and whether they can be achieved will be discussed at the time of consultation.

What Botox won't do for you

It is a common misconception that facial aesthetics is the saviour of all your problems, making your crow's feet, frown lines and wrinkles a distant memory. While this is true to an extent, there are a number of things that Botox treatments won't do for you.

It won't change your lifestyle – having Botox treatments may give you a boost in confidence but it will not change your lifestyle. While we all want a better life, facial aesthetics won't change any relationships you have, won't affect your career or job prospects and won't make you any more money.

It's not permanent – a common misconception for facial aesthetics is that all the procedures are permanent. The truth is the only permanent treatments are surgical; the effects of Botox are temporary and will wear off after about 4–6 months. Facial treatments are not a one off: to maintain your look you need them 3 to 4 times a year.

It won't give you the 'frozen' look – I mentioned before that there is a myth that getting any facial work done will freeze your face completely. Again, this isn't true: Botox will not give you that stiff look so you can still do things like frowning, raising your eyebrows or winking!

It won't improve your mood – there have been no conclusive studies that have proved getting any facial aesthetics treatments will improve your mood.

It won't reverse ageing – it is important that we make sure we look after our skin throughout our lives because there is no turning back the clock to fix it. Botox treatments won't reverse any aging to the skin, including any damage caused by the sun. The treatments received act as way of freezing time to prevent any further ageing or damage rather than reversing it.

Procedure

A very fine needle is used and generally this treatment is not described by most as painful and can be well tolerated with no anaesthetic. Please request an anaesthetic cream or ice if you are nervous about needles.

The aim of Botox treatment is to significantly reduce the movement of the muscles causing expression lines (dynamic lines), specifically the frown and crow's feet; worry lines on the brow may also be treated as an 'off label indication. Successful treatment may not cause the expression lines themselves to disappear completely and it may not 'completely freeze' the expression, particularly if extreme effort is exerted to make an expression.

Botulinum toxin is not suitable for lines present without expression (static lines). Your practitioner will advise you.

Advanced and off-label indications include: horizontal brow lines, lip lines, chin 'poppling', muscles on the lower face and neck, lifting the mouth corners, improving the jaw line and the appearance of the neck. The 'chewing muscle' may also be treated to soften a square jaw or to prevent teeth grinding or jaw clenching at night.

Before treatment – it is important you tell your practitioner about any medicines or dietary supplements you are taking, as some medicines can adversely affect the way the toxin works or increase your risk of bruising.

If you are taking supplements such as Vitamin A, C or E, Gingko Biloba, garlic, fish oils, St. Johns Wort or some pain killing medicines such as aspirin or ibuprofen, then these can increase your risk of bruising and it may be advisable to stop taking them a few days before your treatment. It is also advisable that you do not drink alcohol the night before your treatment, for the same reason.

Make-up will need to be removed prior to the injections and you will be advised not to reapply it for 12 hours in order to reduce the risk of infection or irritation at the injection sites.

Be aware of the necessary after care advice and that your schedule allows for you to follow it.

After treatment – you will be advised to keep the target muscles active for a few hours and to avoid extremes of heat or cold, vigorous exercise, lying down or leaning over for 4-6 hours.

After treatment it is expected that you will start to see an improvement within 2 or 3 days. For some people this takes longer. The full result may be judged at 2-3 weeks. You will be invited to attend a review appointment at 2-3 weeks where the success of the treatment may be assessed and adjustments to your personal treatment plan made, if necessary.

How long will it last? – results tend to last 3-4 months. Movement will begin recovering from 8 weeks. Frequent treatment at intervals of less than 3 months is not recommended. Repeating treatment when movement recovers will deliver optimum results over time. Frequency of treatments may be reduced according to the quality of your skin and your response to treatment.

--

Smoker's lines

Correcting Smoker's Lines with Botox

Do you, or have you ever smoked? If the answer is yes, then you're probably expecting a lecture about how bad smoking is for your lung health, but that's not what I want to talk about; I want to talk about smoker's lines.

Smoking is bad for your skin too, and is a significant contributing factor to the premature ageing of your skin, alongside sun exposure. The effects of smoking start to show after about a decade of the habit, speeding up normal ageing and leading to the early appearance of wrinkles. This is because the nicotine in the cigarettes causes a narrowing of the blood vessels that supply the surface layers of your skin. This reduction in blood flow means that the skin cells don't get as much oxygen or vital nutrients needed to support them and keep them healthy. It's also been shown that many of the other chemicals present in tobacco smoke damage the collagen and elastin found in your skin; these are your skin's support structures, so when they get damaged skin starts to sag and wrinkle.

Finally – I know, it's starting to sound like a lecture, isn't it! – the physical act of smoking, and the facial expressions made, can also lead to the production of certain dynamic wrinkles. As you suck on and inhale from a cigarette, much like a straw, you purse your lips, leading to the formation of straight-line wrinkles in the area surrounding the top and bottom lips; it's usually worse above the top lip, under the nose. After many years of smoking, these lines don't just appear when you smoke, but are present when your face is at rest and you are not moving your mouth. It is these lines which are referred to as characteristic smoker's lines. Similarly, you may also squint your eyes to avoid the smoke as you inhale, and this adds to the formation of crow's feet and frown lines.

All in, being a smoker will lead to you looking old before your time.

Now, of course I would advise you to quit the habit and your NHS GP can help you with solutions to achieve that. What I can also offer is a solution to the premature ageing and wrinkles associated with smoking.

During a face-to-face consultation with me, Dr Harry Singh, at my clinic in Stevenage, Hertfordshire, I can assess your medical and smoking history, current health and the presence of smoker's lines. If botulinum toxin injections are the right solution for you, I can prescribe them as a cosmetic treatment. In my clinic, I like to use the Azzalure™ brand of botulinum toxin; other products include Botox®.

Treating these lines is an advanced technique, so it's important that it is performed by someone with advanced training and experience. As a dentist, I understand the anatomy of the mouth area and have been performing cosmetic injections for over 17 years.

There are three ways to treat these lines:

- toxin only
- dermal fillers only
- combination of both

My criteria for treating with toxin only is if the lines are superficial, worsen when the patient pouts their lips and the patient does not want any fillers to increase the size of their lips. I do warn these patients that we cannot guarantee to eliminate the lines. The toxin is placed very superficially, avoiding the philtrum area and injected close to the vermillion border, the usually sharp edge between the lips and the normal skin. I warn the patient that they may feel numb and find it hard to whistle or say certain letters for a couple of days post-procedure.

Dermal fillers can be used in isolation if the patient's main concerns are the lack of volume in the lips or lack of definition of the vermillion border. There are also some people who simply do not want any toxin treatments.

If the lines are very deep and do not worsen when the patient pouts their lips, I would use a combination of toxin and dermal fillers. The toxin will help relax the muscle and the dermal filler will increase the volume of the lips/borders to help stretch the skin and reduce the appearance of these lines.

In addition to placing fillers in the lip borders and lips themselves, I will also consider using a fine filler to directly 'fill' the smoker's lines. My protocol is to use toxin first and when reviewing, assess whether we need to place a fine filler directly.

I always tell my patients that we cannot guarantee to eliminate the smoker's lines and they may need additional treatments, such as laser skin resurfacing.

--

Sad face

Is your Depressor Anguli Oris (DAO) muscle the reason for your 'frowny face'?

Do people often ask you if '*everything is alright?*', or tell you to '*cheer up*? If so, this could be a sign that you have a reverse or 'upside down' smile, such that the corners of your mouth, even when you are not moving your mouth or lips, have a tendency to point downwards, creating an unhappy look.

The cause of this downwards 'tugging' is an overactivity in one of the many muscles that we use to move our mouth so we can speak, eat and make facial expressions.

The muscle in question is called the Depressor Anguli Oris, or DAO for short. The clue in its name is the word 'depressor', as this is the muscle that is responsible for lowering the corners of the lips and mouth, often used when we wish to express displeasure or repulsion. We have a DAO muscle on each side of the mouth. It is triangular with an anchor at the corner of the mouth and a flat side along the chin. If this muscle is too active, then it can start to tug down on the corner of the mouth even when we aren't calling on its services to make faces. This repeated action can lead to the formation of marionette lines, as the overlying skin is constantly being pulled down by the overactive muscle. As we age, these lines will become more and more pronounced.

Marionette lines are the lines, folds or wrinkles that start from the corners of the mouth and head in a downwards direction, eventually reaching the chin. They get their name from the mouth shape of marionette puppets, or ventriloquists' dummies.

If you try to pull a sad face, you will be able to see and feel the constriction of the DAO muscle at the jawline and can see how strong it is at tugging down the corners of your mouth.

As well as treating deeper lines and wrinkles in this area with dermal fillers, such as the Restylane range which I use in my clinic in Stevenage, Hertfordshire, the DAO can also be relaxed with the use of botulinum toxin injections. This treatment isn't right for everyone, but after a face-to-face consultation, I will be able to diagnose if you have an overactive DAO and if injections with botulinum toxin, on its own, or with dermal fillers would be the most appropriate treatment for you.

Treating the DAO and marionette lines in this way – in fact, any injections of botulinum toxin in the lower face, i.e. below the usual areas of crow's feet and frown lines – is very much an advanced technique and must be performed by someone with significant training and experience. In the wrong hands, complications could arise through incorrect placement of the treatment in the muscles which could have an effect on the positioning of the mouth, lips and teeth, and even affect your ability to bite, chew, suck or talk. That's why it's important to see someone like me: I have been prescribing and performing wrinkle-relaxing treatments of this kind for over fifteen years, plus as a dentist, I am very familiar with the anatomy of the mouth.

--

Gummy smile

How to correct a 'gummy smile' with Botox

A smile is a beautiful thing. It signals an emotional response of joy and happiness, or amusement to those around us. A smile is commonly said to 'light up' someone's face. But sadly, some people don't like their smile, and this isn't always because they don't like their teeth. Some people feel that when they smile they show too much of their gums, usually above their top teeth, or that their gums looks too prominent compared to their teeth – this is referred to as a 'gummy smile', or an 'excessive gingival display', if you want to be technical.

Having a gummy smile can make a person feel self-conscious and less willing to smile, especially in social situations or in photographs, so the beautiful expression of their emotions is stifled. If this is your concern, then keep reading and learn how we can effectively treat this.

When it comes to remedies for a gummy smile, the traditional route, available to dentists and their patients, was fairly invasive and involved a procedure called a 'gingivectomy'. Basically, this is oral surgery to reduce the look of a gummy smile by removing gum tissue. All in, this is costly for the patient, painful and requires time to recover from; it is a radical approach to what is in the main a cosmetic problem. (Gingivectomy is appropriate for some medical and dental conditions, however.)

Thankfully, we now have botulinum toxin products. Most people are familiar with the use of Botox or botulinum toxin as a cosmetic solution for wrinkles such as frown lines and crow's feet, but these anti-wrinkle injections can also be used in all sorts of places, and for various medical problems where muscle spasms cause a variety of conditions.

Following a face-to-face consultation and discussion with me, Dr Harry Singh, I can prescribe Azzalure (a brand name for botulinum toxin) as a solution for reducing a gummy smile. I will ask you to smile and will review your concerns about how much gum is on show. As a dentist I will be able to assess if this option is right for you and we can discuss whether other dental concerns are also affecting your smile and whether these require addressing to create a treatment programme that will give you an effective solution.

The botulinum toxin injections would be used to reduce the strength of certain muscles around your mouth to depress your lips when you smile. In other words, we weaken the muscles a little so your lips do not rise as high above your teeth when you smile. This is achieved by injections of very small doses of Azzalure into four specific points. It's important that you go to an advanced practitioner for treatment like this as they must understand the anatomy of the muscles around the mouth, and the dose of botulinum toxin required to correct the gummy smile but not impact on the general movement of the mouth or your ability to smile, chew, talk, drink, kiss etc.

Treatment for a gummy smile with botulinum toxin is not a permanent solution but will last for approximately 4 to 6 months. You will require regular, repeat treatments to maintain your 'new smile'.

--

Chin

Bothered by a dimply 'golf ball' chin? Find out how to soften it with Botox

The chin is an important area of the face. As well as adding balance to the overall facial profile, achieving markers of beauty and masculinity, it is also involved in the movement and facial expressions made in the mouth area. The chin itself is controlled by one big muscle called the mentalis.

If you try to tighten the area by clenching your chin muscles and pushing out your bottom lip, you will be able to feel the effects of mentalis as the area becomes more solid to the touch and achieves a dimpled appearance and feel, much like the outside of a golf ball.

In some people the mentalis muscle can become hyperactive, or overused, and this can lead to the dimples or wrinkles generated from its dynamic action being visible all the time, even at rest, when they are not tightening the chin. Having visible depressions, roughened skin or deep creases in the chin can make a person look sad, doubtful, disdainful or maybe even angry, when they're not, as these are all emotions where we use the chin to display such feelings. All of this can lead to self-consciousness.

One very unpleasant description of this appearance,

which can affect both men and women, is 'scrotal chin'; not very appealing, I'm sure you will agree! Thankfully, as with treating other hyperactive facial muscles, such as those involved in teeth grinding or squinting, which can cause crow's feet, modern cosmetic medicine has a solution – botulinum toxin injections.

Although botulinum toxin is most commonly used and licenced as an anti-wrinkle treatment it can also be used to treat over-active or spasming muscles. This means we can use it to treat the muscle in the chin to weaken it slightly and reduce the appearance of dimples and wrinkles.

Treating the chin is an advanced technique and should not be done by inexperienced or underqualified practitioners. It is important that you seek out someone with adequate prescribing qualifications, training, experience and understanding of the underlying anatomy and botulinum toxin doses required. Incorrect treatment of this area could lead to over-weakening of the muscles, impacting on jaw movement, and in the worst case, inadvertently affecting your ability to chew properly, or even open and close your mouth.

As a dentist and facial aesthetic practitioner, you can be assured that I am fully qualified to diagnose and prescribe treatment for the chin and mentalis muscle and have a detailed knowledge when it comes to the anatomical structures involved in the mouth and jaw. This means that during a consultation I can advise you whether Azzalure is the right treatment for you based on the concerns that you have and your medical history. Combining other facial aesthetic treatments, such as dermal fillers, may also be an option, depending on the depth of creases around your chin and mouth.

Any treatment with botulinum toxin is not permanent, usually lasting 4 to 6 months before a repeat dose is required to maintain the correction.

--

Neck

"Gobble, Gobble!" Treating a turkey neck with Botox

Ageing is a tricky process that creeps up on us. Most of us start to notice fine lines and wrinkles around our eyes, tell-tale crow's feet, then maybe a frown line or two in between our eyes, all of which signals that our faces are starting to age. You may look at your hands, often regarded as the best way to really know someone's age, but do you ever look at your neck?

Our necks are hard-working parts of our bodies. They must hold up our head, for starters. We stretch them in different directions all day long and they're at the forefront of most of the sun exposure that we get during a lifetime, often not having all the UV sunscreen protection that would be recommended.

This means that over time, the skin on our neck become less smooth, loses volume and suffers from photo-damage in terms of changes to texture, tone and pigmentation. As this happens, the strong muscular bands that do all the work of keeping our heads up, known as platysmal bands, start to show through the thinning skin layers, giving the characteristic 'turkey neck' appearance.

When it comes to ideals of beauty, especially beautiful necks, you can't help but be in awe of the bust of the Egyptian Queen Nefertiti. Granted, we have no actual 'selfies' of the beautiful lady to prove that the artwork done in her name was a genuine representation, but still, it shows what a beautiful, elongated, smooth neck can do for a woman and why Nefertiti was regarded as such a 'goddess'. Given the choice of a turkey neck or having a Nefertiti lift, I think we know what everyone would choose.

Good news then, because at my clinic in Stevenage, Hertfordshire we can reduce the appearance of platysmal bands, restoring a more youthful appearance to the neck, without impacting on function or neck movement, using botulinum toxin injections.

During a consultation, I will ask you to clench your teeth together in an exaggerated smile which allows me to see your neck muscles in full action, as well as how prominent your platysmal bands are at rest, when you are doing nothing. This will allow me to determine if this treatment will be of benefit to you. I will also take a detailed medical history to make sure that you are suitable. Depending on the severity of the lax skin, wrinkles or volume loss in your neck, I may also discuss other aesthetic treatments which can be combined for a more complete solution.

If we go ahead with botulinum toxin treatment it will be injected in very small doses into specific points along the neck muscles. The toxin will take about a week to work and will weaken the muscles ever so slightly, so they become less prominent and improve the appearance of your neck. It's not a permanent solution, as the botulinum toxin does wear off over time, so you will require repeat treatments every 4 to 6 months to maintain the result.

I would rather under-dose and see you again for any necessary top-ups than be over-optimistic on your first visit and overdose, causing complications. By finding a practitioner who will 'baby step' in the lower third of your face you will greatly reduce the risks and be a happier customer.

--

Bruxism

Treating teeth grinding, clenching and a square jaw with Botox

Our jaw is a pretty clever thing. We move it up and down regularly throughout the day as we talk, chew, bite and yawn. It also plays an important role in creating a pleasing and attractive shape to the human face. A wide jaw, which can create a square-shaped look to the lower face, is quite a common occurrence, and although desirable in men as a sign of strength and masculine beauty, it is not considered as attractive in a female.

The appearance of a square jaw is caused by prominent masseter muscles, or chewing muscles. If you place your hands at the ends of your jaw bone, just below your ears, and then clench your teeth together you will feel the masseter muscles as they harden under your fingertips.

In the case of a square jaw, the masseter tend to be excessively active muscles, which means they have become somewhat 'pumped up' through additional exercise, usually as a result of teeth grinding or clenching. The medical name for teeth grinding is bruxism, and it is an incredibly common condition whereby you move your jaw, usually whilst sleeping, and grind the surfaces of your teeth together. This has the effect of wearing down the surface of your teeth, usually corrected through the use of a dental shield at night, but it also exercises your masseter muscles making them more bulky and stronger, leading to the square jaw appearance. Thankfully, we now have a solution to both – botulinum toxin injections. In this case, we would use it to treat the masseter muscle to reduce its activity to more manageable levels.

As a dentist, I am very familiar with the anatomy of the jaw and have encountered many hundreds of patients over the years who regularly grind their teeth in their sleep, so I can advise you during a face-to-face consultation if prescribing botulinum toxin to treat your masseter muscles will both reduce the dental implications of your bruxism, as well as improve the square-like appearance of your jawline, if this is of concern.

Treating the masseter muscles with Azzalure is an advanced technique, so it is important that you see someone with experience, training and understanding of the appropriate dosing required and the effect on the anatomical structures. Seeing an advanced practitioner, like myself, means that you will reduce your risk from over-treatment which could weaken the muscles too much and impact on the movement of your jaw and your ability to bite or chew properly, or even open and close your mouth.

Treatment for a square jaw and bruxism with

botulinum toxin is not a permanent solution but will last for approximately 4 to 6 months. You will require regular repeat treatments to maintain the correction but you should notice a reduction in the dosing required to maintain the muscle activity at a level that helps you to stop grinding your teeth and brings your face back into a more attractive shape.

--

Hyperhidrosis

What is hyperhidrosis?

This means excessive sweating. Sweating is one of the most important ways in which the body loses heat; however, people with hyperhidrosis produce more sweat than needed to control their temperature.

Hyperhidrosis is a common problem for men and women and is estimated to affect 1-2% of the UK population.

If you have ever suffered with anxiety and then had sweaty armpits at an occasion, you will know how upsetting this can be. People with hyperhidrosis suffer with over-sweating most days in winter as well as the summer. Often there is no body odour but just a damp patch that shows up and gets worse the more you think about it. People with hyperhidrosis can produce a large volume of sweat. This means that the hands, feet, chest or armpits (depending on which part of the body is affected) may be constantly damp. This may make normal everyday activities more difficult to carry out and it can cause embarrassment at work or socially. However, it is not true that hyperhidrosis causes body odour; the smell that some people think is due to sweating is in fact caused by bacteria if sweat remains there for a long time

What is the cause of hyperhidrosis?

Although neurologic, metabolic, and other systemic diseases can sometimes cause excessive sweating, most cases occur in people who are otherwise healthy with normal sweat glands. Heat and emotions may trigger hyperhidrosis in some, but many who suffer from hyperhidrosis sweat nearly all the time, regardless of their mood or the weather.

There are two main types of hyperhidrosis:

Focal hyperhidrosis is the more common type involving excessive sweating on the feet, hands and in about 30 – 40% of cases, the armpits.

Generalised hyperhidrosis affects the whole body. It is much less common and is usually caused by another illness such as an infection, diabetes or when the thyroid gland is overactive. The excessive sweating usually stops when the illness is treated.

Examples of triggers include:

- exercise
- heat or cold
- alcohol, coffee or tea, smoking, hot or spicy food
- stress, anxiety or strong emotions

What can I do about hyperhidrosis?

Choose clothing that will keep you cool. Natural fibres are cool, but they absorb sweat and can remain damp; some synthetic fibres are warm but they draw sweat away from the body and feel dry. Consider having a change of clothing available during the day.

Keep your work environment cool and well aired.

Avoid the food and drinks that trigger sweating. These will be different for everyone, but you will probably know what causes problems for you.

Reduce stress, tension and anxiety. These are common problems for everyone, though people with hyperhidrosis have the extra difficulties of coping with sweating. Think about how you can reduce stress during the day, plan your activities carefully and make time to relax.

Pay attention to your personal hygiene. Odour can be reduced by taking frequent showers. Although this will not be convenient for people who constantly sweat it is an effective and simple measure to take.

What treatment is available?

Botulinum toxin treatment is recommended for the treatment of auxiliary hyperhidrosis. When small doses are injected into the skin, it blocks the actions of the nerves that supply the eccrine glands and this prevents the glands from producing sweat. It blocks the nerve endings but over about 6-12 weeks new nerve endings grow to replace them. This means that the effects of treatment last for several months but eventually they will wear off.

What happens during treatment?

Using a very fine needle, your doctor will inject a small amount of a solution into 10 to 15 places about 1cm apart and spread evenly in each armpit. The treatment takes about 30 minutes and you should notice some change for the better within a week of your treatment.

Different people have different responses to treatment. In a clinical trial, sweat production was reduced by 83% one week after treatment. Furthermore, sweating was reduced by at least half in 95% of patients. Your next treatment can be given when the effects of the first course wear off, this usually happens after 4 to 7 months.

--

Five celebs with bad Botox

Like most things in life, there can be too much of a good thing. Many of Hollywood's finest overuse Botox, making their faces appear unnaturally smooth, taut and frozen.

Here are a few examples.

Kim Kardashian – Kim has been a fan of Botox from a relatively young age, hoping to tap into the 'prevention is better than cure' method. But her forehead is unnaturally taut and robs her face of her natural emotions.

Nicole Kidman – it took Nicole years and years to admit to using Botox, despite having a very prominent Botox brow for much of the last decade. She now says she's stopped using it and can finally move her face again. But every public appearance raises a little more scepticism at her line-free face at 51.

Kylie Minogue – Kylie has been open about using Botox and trying 'everything else'. After years of raised eyebrows, some slightly scary expressions, and looking like she was caught in a wind tunnel, Kylie admits to preferring a more natural look and says she won't go near Botox now.

Simon Cowell – at 58, Simon looks unnaturally young and smooth for his age. He was one of the first male celebrities to own up to having Botox and is said to be addicted to the youth-enhancing product, as well as having other surgical procedures.

Tom Cruise – Tom has always denied using cosmetic procedures and actually said he never would. But his appearance has, at times, suggested otherwise with his look garnering comments like "'inflated and puffy" and comparisons to a "hamster in a tuxedo".

4.2 Dermal fillers

Introduction

The popularity of dermal fillers has grown rapidly in recent years because they offer the rejuvenating and enhancing aesthetic improvements previously only achievable with surgery, but at lower cost and with limited-to-no recovery time. According to data from the American Society for Aesthetic Plastic Surgery (ASAPS), more than 1.6 million dermal filler treatments were performed in 2011, making them the second most popular nonsurgical cosmetic procedure performed in the USA after neuromodulators; the latter procedure is frequently performed in concert with dermal filler injections.

As public awareness and acceptance of dermal fillers grows, so does the size of the market, with an estimated 160 products currently available worldwide from more than 50 companies. Their main indications are the filling of rhytides and folds, and correction of soft tissue loss due to disease or age. Increasingly, fillers are used for volume replacement and enhancement procedures, including cheek and chin augmentation, tear trough correction, nose reshaping, midfacial volumisation, lip enhancement, hand rejuvenation, and the correction of facial asymmetry. As the indications and the number of procedures performed increases, the number of complications will likely also increase.

--

Nasolabials

Treating nose-to-mouth lines is simple with dermal fillers

Firstly, I know what you're going to say...what is a nasolabial fold? It's certainly a mouthful of a word, but what it refers to is very simple, and most of us get them, especially as we age. Nasolabial folds, or nose-to-mouth lines, refer to the depressions or grooves that run from the lower corners of the nose, the medical term for which is 'naso', down to the corners of the lips, the 'labia'; hence nasolabial or nose-to-mouth lines.

As simple as they are to define, they are also simple to address by plumping up the area, reducing the mild dip, moderate crease or deep depression, creating a more youthful look with the use of injectable dermal fillers.

Both men and women start to see the appearance of nasolabial lines as they age. This occurs as we lose volume in the cheeks and upper face, which causes sagging in the area and the dropping of the fold of the cheek into the nose area. Dermal fillers can be used very effectively on male and female faces to add back volume and structure to the ageing face in the cheek and nasolabial region.

I use hyaluronic acid-based dermal filler products at my clinic in Hertfordshire. Hyaluronic acid, or HA for short, is a natural component of our skin that our body makes daily. It draws in water to our skin and helps it stay plump and hydrated, which is more youthful looking. Our bodies need to produce lots of HA each day because natural HA doesn't last very long before we metabolise it. Sadly, as we age, we produce less and less natural HA daily; this is why children have such plump faces compared to adults. Scientists have, in the last three decades, discovered ways to manufacture synthetic, longer-lasting HA from non-animal sources, which is perfectly safe to use in humans. I use the Restylane product range which has been clinically proven since the early 1990s for cosmetic use and has one of the longest records for safety and efficacy of any dermal filler brand.

Restylane is non-animal-based and comes in different formulations or 'thicknesses' for use in different areas of the face for maximum benefit. It also comes with built-in local anaesthetic through the addition of lidocaine into the product syringe. This means the area is numbed as it is treated to make it much more comfortable. All the products are temporary, but you can expect the results to last between 6 and 12 months, depending on the severity of your nasolabial lines and which specific product we use to treat them.

How deep the folds are, and the amount of volume loss, will also determine the optimum amount of Restylane syringes I will require to give you the result you are looking for. Your body will still metabolise the HA over time but will do so a lot slower than it does with its natural HA, hence the long-lasting results. You can maintain the correction with repeat treatments at Aesthetics clinic and I will call you back for regular appointments to see how things are looking.

--

Marionette lines

How to treat marionette lines with dermal fillers

Marionette lines are vertical skin folds or wrinkles which start from the corners of the mouth and head in a downwards direction, eventually reaching the chin. They get their name from the mouth shape seen in marionettes, string puppets or ventriloquists' dummies, where a block of wood opens and closes to simulate speech from the mouth.

As we age, marionette lines will get more and more pronounced, eventually creating this puppet-like mouth appearance in older age, yet women and men in their 30s, 40s or 50s will start to notice the appearance of this ageing effect on their faces, as small creases appear at the corners of the mouth. As well as being a sign of ageing, many people dislike these lines as they have the effect of a down-turned smile or 'frowny face', making the individual appear unhappy or sad, even when they are not. This can cause others to comment about their need to 'cheer up' or affect an individual's self-confidence, ultimately having an impact on their mental health and perhaps making their emotions match their face through unhappiness or depression.

Marionette lines coincide with a loss of skin firmness, elasticity and volume in the lower face, combined with the evil that is gravity. Restoring lost volume and structure to the face can help define and support areas of laxity, such as the appearance of lines around the nose and mouth. Genetics (natural ageing), sun exposure and smoking can all cause these lines to appear and get worse, often accelerating the effects. Like many other areas of facial ageing, such as nasolabial or nose-to-mouth lines, marionette lines can be addressed effectively with the use of dermal or soft tissue fillers.

In my clinic in Stevenage, Hertfordshire, I use the Restylane range of hyaluronic acid-based dermal filler products which are temporary, clinically proven and effective. Restylane products were first used in the mid-1990s and were originally developed in Sweden.

I choose this range because they have such a long history of proven science and clinical trial data which shows how safe they are to use in cosmetic treatments; which I have been performing myself for over fifteen years.

Hyaluronic acid-based soft tissue fillers not only contain a synthesised version of a natural substance that our bodies make daily to keep our skin hydrated, but they come in different thicknesses of the hyaluronic acid (HA) gel which means that they have been created to last much longer in the body compared to our natural HA, which we metabolise daily. By placing different thicknesses or gel derivatives from the Restylane range, I am able to add long-lasting volume, definition or hydration to the areas that need it most, to plump out visible folds and depressions. During a consultation we can discuss the extent of your manifestation of marionette lines and the best treatment approach, in terms of the most appropriate type of Restylane product to use, and the quantity or number of syringes needed to achieve the level of correction of the lines at the corners of your mouth. It may be that a combination of aesthetic treatments or products will achieve the best results.

Restylane HA gels normally last between 6 and 9 months before they are completely reabsorbed naturally by your body, giving you a long-lasting result which we can maintain with additional treatments at repeat clinic visits during the year.

--

Lips

From Hollywood Lips to the Essex Lips, it seems that a commonly requested procedure from our aesthetic patients is the non-surgical lip augmentation. Lips have always created attention and there is a high public demand for lip enhancement, which many consider to be a sign of attractiveness.[4] Full and well-defined lips showcase youth, health, attractiveness and sexuality. Wider, fuller and curved lips and a short upper white lip are signs of female attractiveness.[5] We are, of course, also used to seeing with celebrities showcasing their pouts, from Kylie Jenner to Katie Price and most of the *Love Island* cast.

But why do we see so many distorted results? In this section we will look at how you can create the perfect pout. This will involve balancing age-specific treatments with the correct product selection.

Let's start with who is legally allowed to carry out these procedures. Shockingly, anyone can – from your local hairdresser to your local beautician. Dermal fillers are not classified as Prescription Only Medicine (POM), so are freely available to all. However, the enzyme used to reverse dermal fillers, Hyalase, is a POM, so can only be administered by a prescriber or a prescriber must supervise its use.

Anatomy

In Caucasians, the upper lip is narrower, only accounting for 40% of the total volume, with the remaining 60% allocated to the lower lip. A current trend is to increase the upper lip to the same size as the lower lip but this will not look natural. However, in Afro-Caribbeans, the split is 50:50.

Let's take a look at the most salient features of the perfect pout.

- The skin above the vermillion border is smooth without any visible rhytides.

- There are sharply defined philtrum columns.

- There is a well-defined cupid's bow centrally.

- The upper lip has a prominent philtrum.

- The lower lip has a small depression centrally and two side projections.

- The upper lip projects 2mm further than lower lip.

- The main arterial blood supply is from the

superior and inferior labial arteries (branches of the facial artery). The mental artery supplies the chain and lower lip.[6]

Ageing process

As we age, there are marked differences in the appearance of our lips, such as:

- A loss of fullness and projection
- The development of rhytids
- A reduction of the vermillion border
- An inversion of the lower lip
- A reduction of show of the upper teeth
- An increased show of the lower teeth
- A flattening of the cupid's bow
- A flattening of the philtrum columns
- A lengthening of the cutaneous upper lip
- A reduction of the nasolabial angle
- A reduction in the mentolabial angle
- A reduction in vermillion pigmentation

Please note, there is no actual volume loss, it's just a redistribution of thickness of the lip towards length, loss of elasticity and resulting droopiness.

There are also some age-related dental changes that can cause ageing of the lips. For example, tooth wear affects the smile arc, and tooth loss causes alveolar ridge resorption, resulting in decreased facial height. Dentures will also affect the position of soft tissues and lips.

Complications

As with all procedures there are potential complications. Your practitioner will explain these to you before any treatment begins and will do everything they can to minimise/avoid these complications. If complications do occur your practitioner will know how to manage them.

The soft tissue around the lips is loose, delicate and easily expandable, and the lips have a high muscle activity and rich vascularisation. This means they are highly sensitive to trauma and prone to swelling and bruising. Any injection will cause oedema (swelling) and this will not necessarily be symmetric.

Other common post-treatment side effects include:

Swelling - apply a cold compress

Bruising – arnica cream/ tablets can help, as can eating pineapple, as it contains bromelain, which increases the discharge of metabolic waste

Tenderness and redness – take over-the-counter pain killers

All the above are transient and mild and will self-resolve within one week.

Five things you need to know about lip fillers

Reversible – lip fillers are a reversible procedure that can be removed easily if you aren't happy with the end results or if there are any lumps or bumps. The process is reversed by injecting an enzyme into the lips to break down the filler.

Two types – there are two types of lip treatments you can have. The first is enhancement: this is usually for younger clients who want to improve the foundations of what they already have. The second treatment is restoration: this is for older patients whose lips have thinned out and need to be re-built gradually.

Medical professional – any kind of lip filler treatment must be carried out by a qualified medical professional!

Face shape – the shape of your face will determine how big your lips can be without looking unnatural.

It is recommended that you look at photos to see what suits different face shapes the best. Good examples are people like Angelina Jolie or Kylie Jenner; they have naturally round faces so they can get away with having bigger lips.

Temporary – as with most facial aesthetics, lip fillers are not permanent; they will wear off after 9–12 months so you will need a top-up every year to maintain your luscious lips.

--

Cheeks

All you need to know about cheek fillers for cosmetic enhancement

Well-defined cheek bones and the plump pockets of fat that sit above them are a key facial structure and an important element of what makes a face look beautiful. This area represents a point of beauty in a woman and defines a strong face in a man. As we age, we lose both elasticity in our skin and fat or volume from the face, leading to a less-balanced, less-youthful and undefined facial profile.

This volume loss leads to a loss of cheek fullness and goes on to impact in the direction of gravity to create a sagging jawline and an overall dour look. Augmenting or enhancing the cheeks, in both men and women, can put back the lost volume, instantly raising the face and bringing back a more youthful look. We can achieve this using dermal fillers, which create a more natural improvement in the face than traditional solutions of the past such as surgically-placed cheek implants.

I use hyaluronic acid-based dermal filler products at my clinic in Stevenage, Hertfordshire. Specifically, I use different thickness dermal filler products from the Restylane range which has been clinically proven for cosmetic use since the early 1990s. Restylane products have one of the longest records for safety and efficacy of any dermal filler brands.

So, what is hyaluronic acid? It is a natural component of our skin and we make it daily to aid hydration and keep our skin plump and young-looking. Hyaluronic acid is a natural sponge as it draws in water to an area of tissue. Unfortunately, as we age we produce less and less of our natural hyaluronic acid and this, along with the ageing processes in our skin and fatty layers, results in the loss of volume in our mid-face, or lower and upper cheeks.

Thanks to Restylane, we now have long-lasting, synthetic hyaluronic acid products which are made from non-animal sources and are safe to use in our skin to put back both volume and hydration, where needed. The placement of the hyaluronic acid gel will contour the cheekbone area to bring back that attractive facial profile, whilst also providing lift in the mid-face to correct minor sagging which presents in the jawline. Putting the structural support back into the cheeks with dermal fillers can achieve a significant anti-ageing result, rejuvenating the face.

Restylane comes in different formulations or 'thicknesses' so we can use it in different areas of the face, but also in layers within the skin tissue to achieve different structural support, for maximum benefit. It comes with lidocaine within the syringe, alongside the hyaluronic acid, so has a built-in local anaesthetic to make injections more comfortable.

All Restylane products are temporary, so this is a far cry from permanent dermal fillers or implants, making the products much safer than past solutions. You can expect the results to last between 6 and 12 months, depending on the cheek correction required and which specific product we use to treat the area. The amount of correction needed to address the volume loss in the cheek will also determine the optimum number of syringes of Restylane that are needed to achieve the result you are looking for. Over time your body will naturally metabolise the synthetic hyaluronic acid so long-lasting results can be achieved with regular maintenance treatments to top up the correction.

Jawline

Give yourself the jawline you've always wanted

If you look in the bathroom mirror and the image staring back at you appears to be that of a 'sad-looking' face, complete with wrinkled, sagging or lax skin, then I hate to break it to you, but these are all signs of ageing.

That naughty gravity has an annoying habit of sending everything in a southerly direction as we get older. With our face, this means that as wrinkles start to form, volume and elasticity is lost, and this all heads in a downwards direction. This creates marionette lines from the corners of the mouth to the chin, and a loss of the chiselled, angular line of the jawbone which becomes shrouded with loose skin and small fatty deposits called jowls. The effect of ageing hits both men and women, and ultimately definition is lost along the jawline, but thankfully we have a range of medical aesthetic treatments at Aesthetics in Stevenage, Hertfordshire which can recontour, build volume, redefine and provide lift to the lower face, restoring a more youthful aspect and the jawline you always wanted.

Dermal Fillers

Dermal or soft tissue fillers are a great treatment for adding volume, filling depressions, folds, lines and wrinkles, as well as creating shape and structure, which is exactly what we want to achieve when redefining the jawline.

Using a non-animal, hyaluronic acid gel, which is a temporary injectable, gives the best results. As a dentist and aesthetic practitioner, I have been carrying out treatments with the Restylane® range since 2002 and I love the flexibility that products such as Lyft, Volyme and Defyne give me to define, volumise and hydrate the jawline. The best thing about it is that hyaluronic acid is a natural component of our own bodies, which we produce daily. As we age, we produce less of it, which leads to the loss of hydration in our skin and deeper tissue. By using hyaluronic acid in differing gel thicknesses, which lasts for 6 to 9 months (and in some cases, 12 months), we can rebuild what ageing is taking away. The Restylane products also come with added lidocaine which is a local anaesthetic, meaning that every injection is comfortable.

Botulinum Toxin

Botulinum toxin, most commonly known as Botox®, is a prescription only medicine that can be used to treat lines and wrinkles on the face, but also has many other applications which are less familiar to most people. I use a brand called Azzalure®, and it can be used to treat various areas of the lower face to help bring back jawline definition. Because it's a prescription only medicine, you will need to come to a face-to-face consultation with me, so we can discuss if you are suitable for treatment. Azzalure can be used to reduce activity in the Depressor Anguli Oris (DAO), which drags the corners of the mouth downwards towards the chin, and in the chin itself to reduce a so-called 'scrotal chin' whereby an overactive chin muscle creates dimpling. It can also be used in the masseter or chewing muscles to stop teeth grinding, and to soften a square or wide jaw, which is often unattractive in a female.

Silhouette Soft Threads

Addressing volume loss and overactive muscles will have a significant effect on reshaping the jawline, but to really achieve a long-lasting result against gravity, we need to consider treatments that offer a lifting action. One of the best for this is the Silhouette Soft Thread Lift, sometimes referred to as a puppet face lift. Silhouette Soft Threads are made from Poly-L-Lactic Acid (PLLA) with small cones made from lactic and glycolic acid along their length, separated by knots. These cones are therefore free-floating and bi-directional, acting as little hooks and anchors when the thread is placed into the skin and pulled upwards into position. The PLLA has a stimulatory effect in the skin over time and this makes the body produce new collagen to support the lift, even after the original thread has been dissolved by the body. This will last for 18-24 months and is a great lift for younger women who are not ready for a surgical face lift.

--

Chin

Chin up! Treatments for chin rejuvenation

Whether you are bothered by a weak chin, a dimpled chin or a double chin, there are treatments that can be combined to redefine your chin to the prominence you desire.

Many of us by-pass the chin when we think about the beauty and definition of the face, focussing instead on lips, cheeks and eyes, yet the chin is a vital component that creates facial proportions considered optimal for beauty. Mathematical balance is important, so imperfections in the chin can throw a spanner in the works.

Being concerned about the cosmetic appearance of your chin is an issue for both men and women, and treatment can be tailored equally to produce a strong and appropriately contoured look to the area to suit both the female and male face.

At my clinic in Stevenage, Hertfordshire, I offer many treatment options specifically aimed at improving the area of and around the chin. A combined approach is commonplace in facial aesthetic treatments as it provides a more targeted option aimed at optimising results and providing the most effective solutions to volume loss, overactive muscles, stubborn fat and lax tissue.

Chin fillers

In some people the chin simply doesn't protrude far enough outwards from the face; this is known as a weak or recessive chin. This means there is no clear definition between the chin and the neck, which can make the mouth and lips look out of proportion. Using the Restylane range of hyaluronic acid (HA) based dermal fillers, I can build volume and shape into the chin. The natural enhancement will last between 6 and 9 months, as the body will naturally metabolise the HA over time, so you will require repeat treatments to maintain the desired look.

Scrotal chin

Dimpling on the chin, likened to the bumps that you see on the outside of a golf ball, or, less flatteringly, a 'scrotal chin', can be troublesome if they are present even when no muscle contraction or facial expression is being made. The cause of the dimples is over activity in a muscle called mentalis. This means that the dimples which would usually only appear when the chin is moved by mentalis are present all the time, as deep wrinkles or creases or visible depressions and craters. To reduce the action of this muscle, we can use botulinum toxin injections, perhaps in combination with dermal fillers to treat the deeper wrinkles and folds. Specifically, I use a brand called Azzalure™, but you may also have heard of Botox®. The use of botulinum toxin is a prescription only medicine, so first we will need to have a face-to-face consultation so I can diagnose the over activity in the mentalis and decide if Azzalure treatment is appropriate. Botulinum toxin treatment lasts about four months before the reduction in muscle activity is restored, so repeat treatments are needed to maintain the reduction in wrinkling of the chin.

Double chin

Ageing often leads to small, stubborn pockets of fat in places we'd rather not have them, and a double chin is a very common concern for both men and women as they get older. A double chin is a combination of the extra fatty tissue alongside sagging skin which has lost its elasticity. Injection lipolysis with Desoface provides a great solution to essentially melt the fat cells, allowing them to be flushed out naturally by the body. Desoface uses an ingredient called sodium deoxycholate (deoxycholic acid) which breaks down the fat cells, allowing them to expel their lipid contents. Multiple treatment sessions are needed, and the results will develop over a few weeks as the body flushes out the lipids and the overlying skin starts to tighten up again.

--

Temples

What are temple fillers and why do we use them to correct facial volume loss?

Wondering where your temples are? You're probably not the only one, as it is an area of the face that doesn't get discussed too much, especially when it comes to cosmetic enhancements.

The temples — yes, there are two of them, one on either side of your face — are the small flat areas that you will find if you place your fingers just above your crow's feet area, in line with the tops of your ears, and just below where your forehead starts.

The temporal region, as it's medically called, is quite bony, with little volume in terms of fat compared to, say, the cheeks, where you can pinch a good amount of tissue if you try. Yet as we age, the temples start to lose the small amount of volume they have, and this affects the overall appearance and youthful aspect of the face.

A youthful face is round or oval, with a 'full' appearance to the shape. As we age, the overlying tissue and the bone density of the skull changes and this leads to a loss of this fullness. The easiest way to explain this is that the face goes from a round or oval shape to a 'monkey-nut' appearance, with a distinct concavity or dent in the shape of the face. This changes the face from a youthful appearance to a more skeletal, aged look.

Correcting the hollowing of the temples caused by this volume loss can be done with dermal fillers, the same products often used to augment lips, recontour the jawline, plump up cheeks and correct nose imperfections non-surgically. However, the temple area is also considered to be one of the more complex areas of the face where a good knowledge of the underlying anatomy is paramount, so any practitioner performing temple fillers should have advanced training and experience. I use hyaluronic acid-based dermal filler products at my clinic in Stevenage, Hertfordshire and have been performing cosmetic injectable treatments, including advanced techniques, for over fifteen years.

Usually, adding dermal filler products to the temples will not be a stand-alone process, but part of an overall facial rejuvenation treatment. The temples also affect the structure around them so adding volume back, which will return the roundness of the face, can have secondary effects such as lifting the side of the brow area and can also lessen other changes in the lower face affecting the cheek and nose-to-mouth (naso-labial) lines. Often overlooked, you may be surprised to discover how much difference can be achieved with some hyaluronic acid gel to the temporal region.

Hyaluronic acid (HA) is a natural component of human skin and something that our body makes daily. Our bodies need to produce lots of HA because it acts as a natural moisturiser, drawing in water to our skin to keep it plump and hydrated, but our natural HA doesn't last very long before we metabolise it and then need to make more. Unfortunately, as we age, we are not able to produce as much HA as we did in our youth, so skin becomes dehydrated and less plump. Some clever scientists have synthesized HA from non-animal sources so it is safe for use in humans, the difference being that the injectable HA is made into a longer-lasting gel, so it stays within the tissue for much longer than our natural hyaluronic acid.

I use the clinically-proven Restylane range of dermal fillers which has been proven to be safe and effective since the early 1990s. Restylane comes in different HA gel 'thicknesses' for use in different areas of the face to achieve maximum volume replacement and contouring. It also comes with the local anaesthetic lidocaine for a more comfortable treatment. By using these products in the temporal region, as well as other areas which could benefit from rejuvenation and volume correction, you can expect an improvement in your facial appearance to last between 6 and 12 months. We can then come up with a bespoke treatment plan to maintain the correction with future appointments at Aesthetics in Stevenage, Hertfordshire with me, Dr Harry Singh.

Chapter 5: Skin

5.1 Good skin

5.2 Sun Damage

5.3 Myths about Moisturisers

5.4 Cosmeceuticals

5.5 Sunekos

5.6 Threads

5.1 Good skin

10 simple steps to a more youthful and healthier complexion

Make-up and creams can only cover up unhealthy skin; it is impossible to completely hide it. Healthy glowing skin comes from the inside out. Here are 10 simple steps to achieve this goal.

1. Change your perceptions of ageing

Rather than being anti-ageing, we like to focus on *good ageing*. Do not believe the hype around reverse ageing. Be proud of your age. By following some simple tips, you will feel more confident about your age because your skin will be healthy and glowing. It's all about looking good and feeling great.

> *"I think I am going to love ageing.*
> *But then, what choice is there?"*
> *Angelina Jolie.*

2. Restful sleep

Sleep is important for tissue renewal and overall health. Try to relax before going to bed, e.g. read, or take a warm bath. Eat no later than 2-3 hours before bedtime. Noise is one of the most common sleep disruptions – wear ear plugs to muffle external sounds. Go to bed at the same time every night, whenever possible.

3. Lovingly nurture your body through healthy food

We need the right quantities of nutrients, vitamins and minerals from a wide range of sources, such as grains, fruit and vegetables, nuts, beverages and oils. Ensure you are eating the right types of food at the right time of the day, and that you are having the right balance of protein, carbohydrate and fibre.

4. Use the correct skin care products

At aesthetics we only use natural purified products that have medical evidence behind them. This consists of a three-stage process – stimulate, correct and protect.

5. Sun protection

Vitamin D from the sunshine is essential for the health of your skin; however, too much sunlight is harmful to your skin. A tan is a sign that the skin has been damaged. The damage is caused by ultraviolet (UV) rays in sunlight. However, even when it's not sunny your skin still needs constant protection.

6. Regular exercise

Exercising can contribute to your skin's health. If you're tired, stressed, malnourished, or unable to exercise, it's reflected in the tone, colour and condition of your skin. Luckily, the opposite is also true. That's why your skin is said to 'glow' when you're terrifically happy and healthy.

7. Eliminating toxins

Your skin needs to keep well hydrated, since the human body is 80% water. You can keep hydrated by drinking water, beverages (not coffee, which will dehydrate your skin) and certain foods. Smoking depletes your body of essential nutrients, like vitamin B and C. It also has a dehydrating effect which can make you look older than you are.

Excess alcohol causes dehydration; you can still enjoy a drink, but in moderation.

8. De-stress

Undue stress can cause the adrenal glands to over-stimulate and this can affect your immune system, causing certain skin complaints. Find a way of destressing - fresh air, exercise and relaxation, for example.

9. Love

We all have people who care about us and people

who mean a lot to us. Spend time with these people and you will always have a positive focus.

10. Maintain a youthful mind

You are what you think. Challenge your mind and body at regular intervals and feel the benefits inside and out.

5.2 Sun Damage

Everyone loves a holiday in the sun or nice day sun bathing in the park. It feels good and is in fact necessary in order to receive proper amounts of Vitamin D. However, there is a safe way to achieve a little sun without over-burdening the body with excess free-radical damage and Ultra Violet (UV) radiation.

UVA has been found to cause premature ageing and is present all the time, even on cloudy days. UVB causes burning and is present on sunny days.

The following explains the best ways to protect yourself from the avoidable sun damage that each of us receives on a daily basis as well as the safest ways to obtain some rays.

First, what exactly does Sun Protection Factor (SPF) mean? SPF refers to a sunscreen's ability to absorb UV rays or a sun block's ability to reflect them. They are measured by timing how long it will take for the skin to burn when covered with a sunscreen or block compared to unprotected skin.

For example, SPF 15 means it will take 15 times longer for skin to burn with protection than without it.

Sun Protection Factors range from 2 to 60, but in

reality, an SPF of 30 only protects the skin 4% more than an SPF 15. This is because an SPF 15 absorbs 93% of the UV rays, while an SPF of 30 absorbs 97%. The Department of Health's sun safe advice recommends people use a broad spectrum sunscreen SPF 15 or higher in conjunction with other protective methods.

Additionally, the protection intended from an SPF of any sort is dependent on factors like the amount used and how it is applied, when it is used and how often it is reapplied, and what level of SPF is used and whether it is a screen or a block.

Applying sun protection and general guidance

The amount of product needed to actually receive the amount of SPF intended by the manufacturer is 30 ml to 60 ml, or 6 teaspoons for each appendage, and about half of that for the face.

Application should be much like that of painting a wall. Two coats are always better than one.

When going out into direct sunlight, always apply sunscreen at least 30 minutes beforehand.

And remember, the rays that are most damaging to our DNA and cause premature ageing are the UVA rays. These are present even when it is cloudy and raining outside. So, always apply SPF to your face on a daily basis.

Reapplication should be done every two hours if in direct sun and at least once a day for daily maintenance. This can be achieved either by using a mineral base make-up or a spray sun block.

Stay in the shade between 11am and 3pm and don't rely on sunscreen alone.

Wear clothes that cover your arms and legs, and a wide-brimmed hat.

Wear sunglasses that block UV light to protect your eyes.

Never burn, as sunburn causes permanent damage.

Lastly, and most importantly, which is better, a sunscreen or a sun block?

There seems to be a lot of confusion around this topic; however, it becomes quite simple when we come from a standpoint of chemicals versus non-chemicals and absorbing UV rays rather than reflecting them. A sunscreen uses chemicals as a way of absorbing the UVB rays. These are responsible for our skin's ability to tan (a tan, by the way, is a sign of injury that the skin creates to protect skin cells from DNA damage). Furthermore, if the sunscreen says 'broad spectrum', then it also absorbs UVA rays.

So, if you can't trust sunscreens, can you trust a sun block? Because a sun block reflects the UV rays up and away from the skin, allowing for very little penetration, and also avoids the use of synthetic chemicals, the answer is easy. Ingredients like micronized titanium dioxide, micronized zinc oxide and zirconium oxide are all natural minerals that are non-irritating and will block out both UVA and UVB rays.

Additionally, because they are not chemicals dependent on a time frame, it is only when they are washed off the skin either by sweat or water that they become ineffective. Hence, they provide even longer protection than a sunscreen can! And if texture and thickness is a problem, new formulations using mineral blocks have been developed that are lightweight and do not leave a whitish appearance on the skin.

5.3 Myths about moisturisers

Does 'moisturising' come as second nature to you? Is this habit a good or bad one?

The media and advertising geniuses have certainly done a good job at convincing us that moisturising is a good habit. Catchy marketing slogans like 'botanical hydration', 'firming and wrinkle defying' and 'rich and creamy' have appealed to the vast majority of us as we run to buy the latest over-the counter miracle cream. Unfortunately, the majority of these creams cannot live up to their claims. The truth is, packaging and marketing is most of what your money goes towards rather than the correct ingredients.

Why do we religiously apply moisture cream?

If you suffer from dry and sensitive skin, the answer is tri-fold. First, the continual use of moisturisers has left your skin dependent and addicted to emollients. Next, the ingredients contained in your moisturisers are more often than not causing mild irritation and disrupting the lipid barrier of the skin. All this, combined with an improper diet and environmental factors, has a detrimental impact on your skin. It can no longer produce enough sebum oil and is devoid of the necessary components for repair. Applying a moisturiser can alleviate the feeling of dry and sensitive skin but you are not treating the root cause - the moisturiser itself!

Here comes the science bit.

The rate at which normal skin produces new cells ranges anywhere from a 30–40-day cell turnover cycle.

When the lipid barrier is functioning normally your skin is resilient and well hydrated. However, when skin is continually covered by an occlusive or emollient this cycle can take twice as long, leaving the skin compromised and unable to carry out normal functions like exfoliation and lipid production.

This has three main effects on the skin:

1. Natural barrier function shuts down;

2. Increased dryness and sensitivity;

3. Prematurely ageing skin.

We cannot remember what our skin felt like before the use of moisturisers. We forget that dry skin and sensitive skin is DAMAGED SKIN. If you continue to use moisturisers, you are treating damaged skin with the exact product that caused the dryness and sensitivity in the first place.

Manufacturers have further wreaked havoc on our delicate skin by way of the ingredients used in their 'miracle' creams. Nearly every moisturiser on the market contains some form of irritating or comedogenic ingredient. Check your moisturiser against a list of known irritants and comedogenics. Propylene glycol, glycolic acid, mineral oil, petrolatum, talc, lanolin, parabens and sulphites are just a few of the ingredients that will either clog the skin's pores or bring about inflammation.

Other factors to consider?

Harsh weather conditions and the sun can certainly have their way with our skin if we are not careful. The sun is amongst one of our most harsh and unforgiving skin-harming culprits. Next in line is our daily lifestyle. Smoking, alcohol, stress and a diet lacking in whole fruits and vegetables promotes free-radical damage and eventual premature ageing. Not even the mightiest of moisture creams can reverse that.

How can I protect and prevent inflammation and damage to my skin?

The first step is to discontinue the use of moisturisers. Allow your skin to return to equilibrium. This means the function of your natural skin barrier will return and your skin can exfoliate and shed properly again. This is achieved by using active and simulating ingredients, like L-retinol, that will communicate at the molecular level of the skin for repair and rejuvenation.

Most importantly, do not forget to protect the skin from sun.

5.4 Cosmeceuticals

'Cosmeceuticals' are topical products that provide enhanced skincare benefits that go beyond traditional cosmetics known primarily for covering, moisturising and cleansing the skin. Cosmeceuticals do not have the same regulatory requirements as prescription skincare products and generally lack rigorous clinical trials to substantiate efficacy, potency, or consistency. Cosmeceuticals for skin rejuvenation are now the fastest growing segment of the multibillion-dollar skin care market. Increasingly, cosmeceuticals are being used in professional practices as adjuncts to in-office procedures and prescription drugs as well as stand-alone home treatments.

Patients frequently seek advice from skin care professionals. More scientific studies are being performed on non-prescription topical skincare products and this provides clinicians with more evidence with which to recommend skincare products.

The subject matter can be confusing for both the patient as well as the provider. For the patient, the market offers products that claim the same aesthetic benefits from different combinations of ingredients at discount (low) or premium (high) prices. For the provider, many have had limited formal education on the topic.

Consequently, it can be difficult to sort through the large number of products available to identify those with scientific data to support their efficacy. Of practical concern, discussing and recommending topical skincare products with patients in the midst of a busy clinic can be time consuming. In addition, physicians who are not yet confident in their knowledge of skincare product alternatives may feel awkward when patients ask for recommendations. As a result, many physicians avoid actively discussing cosmeceuticals with patients. This leaves the patient without informed recommendations from their trusted clinician, and uneducated as to how skincare programmes may fit into their overall skin health practices.

Is your skin better? Let me tell you about the new skincare revelation to arrive in Hertfordshire, skinbetter science®

Are you looking for an effective skincare regime that will improve your skin tone, texture, ageing and pigmentation concerns, but haven't got the time to devote to fiddly, time-consuming rituals? Then **skinbetter science®** is just the answer for you, and I'm really pleased to say that it is now available at

Aesthetics clinic in Stevenage, Hertfordshire.

Like many of my aesthetic clients, I'm a busy person, which often leads to me being time poor. I want results, good results, in everything I do, with every minute of my day, which is why I was attracted to the benefits of **skinbetter** as a professional skincare system to offer to you.

skinbetter provides an uncomplicated approach to skincare whilst being scientifically advanced to achieve real results. Many people struggle to follow strict, multi-step skincare routines. The tedium of a step-by-step process doesn't readily fit into most people's lives; this leads to a lack of commitment and before you know it you're not getting the results you want, but you haven't the time to spend in front of a mirror applying one serum followed by another, plus a cream and a sunblock, then repeating the same routine every morning and night.

skinbetter can deliver remarkable results with a single product; but adding in one or more additional products can make a real difference to your skin health without making an onerous demand on your time! Fitting into your real life, the application of your product mix becomes quick and simple and part of your daily routine, rather than a daily chore.

You will not find this range on the high street; the exceptional wealth of active ingredients available in the products can only be dispensed by a medical aesthetic clinic, where your skin health can be properly assessed, and the product choices optimised and recommended just for you.

skinbetter products work on four different levels, allowing an optimal product choice to 'refresh', 'rejuvenate', 'transform' and 'protect' your skin. What could be easier!

Primary focus for discussion with me, your aesthetic practitioner, starts with the Rejuvenate selection of face, eye and neck products which include innovative ingredients including hyaluronic acid, alpha hydroxy acids (AHAs), glycolic acid, peptides, retinoids and lactic acid (in their specialised ingredient, AlphaRet) to rejuvenate and re-texture the skin, and improve the appearance of fine lines and wrinkles. Rejuvenate is preceded by Refresh products which are ideal for cleansing, exfoliating and moisturising your skin. Think of them as preparation products, akin to a wash and scrub before you apply the all-important advanced rejuvenation products. If you're looking for a boost for your skin, then you can consider adding a Transform product to offer immediate lifting-like effects, whether with a quick three-minute mask to reduce lines and wrinkles or a daily refreshing eye gel. These are the pick-me ups of the **skinbetter science** range.

Finally, and most important is to Protect your skin, with an award-winning antioxidant product containing 19 antioxidant ingredients that act as a shield against oxidative stress. Acting as your built-in ninja warrior against marauding free radicals, this will defend your skin from attack whilst you get on with your day, helping to fight off ageing and skin redness.

5.5 Sunekos

Have you heard of Sunekos for rejuvenating your face?

Ageing presents in many ways on the face and isn't just limited to lines and wrinkles or a loss of elasticity to the skin. As we age, skin will lose tone, becoming dry and uneven in texture, perhaps feeling rough. Skin can also suffer from changes in pigmentation or photo-damage which creates uneven patches of skin colour, or age spots, as well as dark under-eye circles. Exposure to sun is partly to blame but genetics, lifestyle choices and the natural pathway of getting older all play a part.

This means that as well as addressing deeper lines and wrinkles with dermal fillers or relaxing dynamic wrinkles, such as frown lines or crow's feet, with botulinum toxins to allow the skin to recover, it's important to consider treatments that can help to restore the whole of the skin, rejuvenating and stimulating the building blocks of new skin.

Sunekos is a new cosmetic injectable product, which, like the Restylane® dermal filler range that I use, contains hyaluronic acid. But what makes Sunekos special is the patented formula of amino acids, which is added alongside the hyaluronic acid to create the injected product. This potent mix of amino acids, which includes glycine, L-proline, L-leucine, L-lysine

HCI, L-valine and L-alanine, helps to regenerate the Extra Cellular Matrix (ECM) – the building blocks which help to make the wall – by stimulating fibroblasts, or skin cells, to produce new collagen and elastin, repairing and rebuilding skin. This process is referred to as dermal biogenesis, literally skin regeneration.

Hyaluronic acid (HA) is a natural component of our skin which draws in water to act as a natural moisturiser, keeping skin hydrated and plump, both of which are signs of youthful skin. HA is made by our bodies daily, but, as we age, we produce less natural HA and our skin suffers in appearance because of this. Amino acids are made by our bodies and are essential for the creation of healthy skin, acting as the precursors to the formation of new collagen and elastin.

Sunekos offers two different treatment options for skin regeneration, which can be performed separately or in combination – Sunekos 200 and Sunekos 1200.

Sunekos 200 contains a low molecular weight HA and Sunekos 1200 is a medium molecular weight HA. The former can be used alone to treat the face, neck, décolletage and hands and is great for younger people. If additional 'cushioning' is required in the case of lax, sagging skin or deeper lines and wrinkles, then Sunekos 1200 can be combined to give extra scaffold support for the dermal biogenesis.

Clinical trials have shown that hyaluronic acid products on their own can cause biorevitalisation in the skin, stimulating fibroblasts. The addition of the amino acids is like adding extra fuel to a fire: their presence stimulates and directly targets the ECM fibroblasts, which is important when it comes to rebuilding the dermal layers of the skin. Participants in trials reported improvements in wrinkles, skin plumpness and hydration, as well as a lifting effect.

I recommend a course of three to four weekly treatments to achieve the best results with Sunekos 200, followed by a repeated course of treatments every six months. If extra support is required with Sunekos 1200, then this will be injected a few days before treatment commences with Sunekos 200. You will start to notice the effects of treatment after a week or so as skin begins to rejuvenate.

5.6 Threads

The Puppet Face Lift with Silhouette Soft Threads

Mention the words 'face lift' and everyone starts thinking about scalpels, cutting into skin and then pulling back on the face, but what about a non-surgical face lift?

Times have changed, and we now have many more options in medical aesthetics that allow practitioners to work with a patient to produce the cosmetically-enhanced results which once could only be achieved with surgery. Surgery still has a place for those with considerable ageing and skin laxity, but if you're not quite there yet, then we can do wonders with thread lifting or a 'puppet face lift'.

The puppet face lift is a term coined, probably by the media I think, to refer to a thread lifting technique with Silhouette Soft Threads to achieve a non-surgical form of face lifting.

The Silhouette Soft Threads are lengths of suture material containing Poly-L-Lactic Acid, or PLLA. Along each thread, which varies in size depending upon where it will be used, are small 'cones' made from lactic and glycolic acids. These cones are separated by knots along the suture line to stop them from sliding up and down the thread but keeping them free-floating between the knots. The cones are bi-directional, which means that from the centre of the thread either 4, 6 or 8 cones will go in each direction out towards the end of the threads. The cones are the anchors for the threads so that when a thread is implanted in the skin, pulled and tightened into place, the cones secure themselves to maintain the lift. Threads are inserted using a fine needle through an entry and exit point. The same entry point will be used for multiple threads, which are usually laid out in a pattern to achieve the designed amount of lifting needed. Treatment takes about 30 minutes and can be used along the jawline, the mid-face and the neck.

These threads are full re-absorbable, meaning they do not remain permanently in the body but dissolve over time, usually after a year. PLLA has a stimulatory effect on the skin tissue, so as well as providing mechanical lifting and skin tightening when the thread is put into position, it also increases the production of the body's natural collagen around the thread for a longer-term result. Known as a foreign body reaction, the presence of the thread tricks the body into making more collagen so the lift from the thread remains in the natural tissues after the PLLA has dissolved.

Due to the nature of the procedure, it's important you only seek treatment from an experienced medical practitioner who has undergone manufacturer-approved training, specifically in the placement of

Silhouette Soft Threads.

Thread lifting with Silhouette Soft is ideal for women and men aged between their mid- to late-30s and their mid-50s, who have a good underlying skin structure but who are showing some slight sagging in the cheeks and jawline, consistent with the early signs of ageing. Such individuals would not yet be candidates for surgical intervention but would benefit from tissue lifting and tightening to improve the laxity. Results of a puppet thread lift last between 18 months to 2 years and treatment can be combined with other aesthetic treatment options such as dermal fillers.

What are the components of Silhouette Soft®?

Silhouette Soft® components are natural and fully absorbable. Polylactic acid, or PLA, has been used for many years in various pharmaceutical and medical applications, such as suture thread, orthopaedic pins, screws and nails for bone fractures, etc. It is also used in new biodegradable stent trials.

Can Silhouette Soft® be used in complete safety?

The development of Silhouette Soft® is based on six years of experience in suture suspension with cones used in reconstructive surgery and cosmetic surgery in the United States (Silhouette Lift®).

Silhouette Soft® is made in Michigan in the USA and is subject to numerous sanitary controls.

Silhouette Soft® received CE 0499 approval and the ISO 13485 standards are in accordance with European Directive 93/42.

How long do the results last?

The visible benefits of Silhouette Soft® treatment can last up to 18 months.

Which areas can be treated?

Silhouette Soft® can be used to treat various parts of the face: contour, lower jaw, and cheeks and cheekbones.

What must be done before Silhouette Soft® treatment?

No special preparation is required prior to Silhouette Soft® treatment.

However, we recommend that you discuss your expectations and ask your doctor any questions you have before starting treatment. Inform the doctor of any treatment you have already received and of any medicines you are currently taking.

Who can provide Silhouette Soft® treatment?

Only doctors thoroughly trained in Silhouette Soft® sutures are authorised to implement the treatment.

What happens immediately after Silhouette Soft® treatment?

After Silhouette Soft® treatment, as with any cosmetic treatment, some slight swelling, redness or bruising may sometimes be observed, but these disappear within days.

There is sometimes a slight wrinkling of the skin (required for optimisation of the treatment) which disappears very quickly. If you experience any side effects, talk to your doctor.

Are there any contraindications to Silhouette Soft® treatment?

You must not use Silhouette Soft® if you are allergic to any of its ingredients.

Is Silhouette Soft® treatment painful?

No, the treatment is performed under local anaesthetic of certain points of the area to be treated, thus avoiding pain during insertion of the suture.

Are there any recommendations to be followed after Silhouette Soft® treatment?

During the week following treatment, do not undergo any dental surgery, and avoid facial massages or any beauty treatment.

For the first few weeks, avoid any contact sport.

It's preferable that you sleep on your back.

In the event of pain, take a pain reliever according to your doctor's prescription.

Chapter 6: Body

6.1 Fat dissolving

6.2. Cellulite

6.3. IV vitamins

6.1 Fat dissolving

Desobody, the latest in fat dissolving injections

Okay, hands up who's got a little bit of wobbly fat here and there which will just not go? We all have, haven't we? I know I have!

No matter how good our best intentions are to eat well and exercise, spending hours and hard-earned money on kale smoothies and gym visits, stubborn pockets of fat remain in areas such as love handles or bra rolls, muffin tops around the tummy, saddle bags on the outer thighs and other areas around the male and female abdomen. It can be very disheartening, for both men and women, when they just won't shift!

Let me tell you more…

Treatment with injection lipolysis

Desobody is a product used for a treatment called injection lipolysis. Lipolysis literally means fat-dissolving and that is what the injection of Desobody into targeted areas will do over a course of treatments. The active ingredient is sodium deoxycholate (deoxycholic acid) which is a special medical detergent that breaks down fat cells. Desobody has a concentration of 1.25% sodium deoxycholate.

There is also another product called Desoface, which

has a lower concentration of sodium deoxycholate (0.5%) for treating double chins.

Treatment with Desobody uses a thin cannula (non-sharp needle) which is placed under the skin through a single insertion point. This means that we can evenly deliver the active ingredient in a fan-like pattern across the whole area where we are wanting to dissolve the fat cells. The amount of Desobody needed will depend on the size of the area(s) being treated. Each session will take around 45 minutes, with only mild discomfort as a local anaesthetic is used to numb the area. Following treatment, you can expect some redness and swelling as the product gets to work on disrupting the fat cells so they release their contents. There may also be some bruising and mild to moderate pain in the first 24-72 hours, which can be managed with over-the-counter pain medications like paracetamol. Over the coming weeks your body will slowly metabolise and expel the released lipids from the fat cells. Repeat treatment is required, and, depending on the area being treated, we recommend 2-4 sessions, spaced 4-8 weeks apart, for optimum results and fat reduction.

It's important to remember that this is not a weight-loss solution or slimming aid. The best candidates for treatment are those who have a medium body weight (BMI), who may be just slightly overweight, and have localised fat deposits, i.e. small, specific areas of fat around their back, stomach, hips, buttocks, inner and outer thighs or knees.

Following completion of the treatment, you can expect the area of fat targeted to be reduced and the firmness of the overlying skin to also be improved.

Treatment with intralipotherapy

Localised fat deposits are subcutaneous adipose tissue accumulations in specific anatomical areas that alter body silhouette. They are unsightly and unresponsive to the normal signals to activate the metabolism (low-calorie diet, physical exercise). They can be successfully treated with intralipotherapy.

Intralipotherapy is a widely used technique in aesthetic medicine. It uses adipocitolytic solutions, which are solutions containing natural cleansers that cause fat cell lysis.

Using intralipotherapy, the solution is released, parcel-style and evenly, directly into the fat layer, gradually reducing its size. The treatment can be repeated after a suitable period of time.

The solution is slow acting and the gradual action needs time to achieve the treatment aim.

The fat cells in the layer treated with sodium deoxycholate will undergo lysis and then a process of degradation and disposal through the lymphatic system.

Before treatment, it is necessary for the patient to undergo careful examination while standing. The treatment includes injection of the substance directly into the fat layer, using a special needle (intralipotherapy needle). Needle access is limited generally to 1-3 times per area.

It is possible to feel mild to moderate pain during treatment, although this is easily tolerated or ignored. The treatment is followed by slight pain, redness, swelling and bruising. These problems are very frequent, transitory and should be considered a normal consequence of the treatment. If the patient notes anomalous symptoms during the period after treatment, meaning anything not described by the qualified practitioner, they must contact him or her without delay.

Oedema, bruising, and pain in the treated area are extremely frequent (more than 50% of cases) but generally do not limit a normal social life or physical activity.

Containment means (sleeves, girdles etc.), lymph drainage or pressotherapies are strongly recommended for the days after treatment.

It is in any case important to follow the instructions of

the qualified practitioner, which will vary according to each case, based on different factors such as the body area treated, the patient's characteristics and the progress of the post- treatment period.

Post-treatment advice

Avoid Aspirin for pain. Take paracetamol and use a fan (for cold air) if necessary.

Ice can be applied for 5 mins post treatment

Try using compression garments for 2-5 days post treatment.

Nodules can last up to one month. These can be managed.

Bruising is frequent. Avoid direct sunlight, sunbeds and heat treatments during your treatment and recovery period.

Do not apply any hot water to the treated area for five days following treatment.

6.2. Cellulite

Treatment for cellulite that works – introducing Celluerase

Plagued by orange peel-looking skin or lumpy, cottage cheese-like bumps on your thighs? Well, you're not alone. The appearance of cellulite is one of the primary dissatisfactions for most women. Many will spend thousands of pounds and hours of their lives trying to alleviate it with creams, massage devices, brushes and compression pants, none of which work.

First things first, what is cellulite and how do you get it?

It's a myth that having cellulite is just due to being overweight. It's true that if you are carrying a few too many pounds, the cellulite will stand out more and be more obvious, but cellulite has a lot to do with genetics and hormones as well. Even slim, fit women can get cellulite. In fact, it's estimated that between 85-98% of women have some cellulite! This means you are very much not alone if you are worried about it.

The problem for women, and why men rarely, if ever, suffer from cellulite, is all down to the way women store fat and the structure and shape of their fat cells. The orange peel or cottage cheese appearance on the skin of the thighs and buttocks is because the fat cells underneath the skin start to push through the overlaying fibrous, connective tissue, which is characteristic in these areas of the female body. The fibrous tethers mean that as the fat is pushed up, it herniates through the spaces and makes the bumps or dimpled look appear on the outside of the skin. Put simply, imagine an old-fashion'ed string shopping bag with a blancmange inside it and how this would bulge through the air holes in between the bag's strings!

Celluerase is designed to release these fibrous bands to reduce the appearance of the dimpling characteristic of cellulite. It is a minimally invasive procedure which must be performed under local anaesthetic, which numbs the area to avoid discomfort. We can treat multiple areas at once, e.g., thighs and buttocks, and only one treatment session is usually required to achieve the desired result. Celluerase can be combined with other active ingredients such as mesotherapy or injectable lipolytic products to help break down the fat and aid lymphatic drainage, to produce a smoother appearance to the skin in the treated area. The lymphatic drainage in the thighs and buttocks is often sluggish so we can use a combined treatment approach to help the body to flush out the area and detoxify. Because this is a minimally invasive treatment, you can expect a little downtime and bruising, but the results you will achieve are significantly better than you will ever get by slathering on expensive creams or rubbing a brush up and down your thighs in the shower every day!

6.3. IV vitamins

What is Intravenous Nutrition Therapy?

IV nutritional therapy is a procedure by which vitamins, minerals, amino acids and other nutrients are slowly administered via a small needle into the patient's vein.

When nutrients are delivered intravenously, the digestive system is bypassed and 100% nutrient absorption is achieved. Introducing nutrients intravenously directly into the circulation ensures that your cells can easily obtain the nutrients needed to repair, heal, function and maintain optimal health.

The anticipated benefits of IVNT include:

- The injectable nutrients are not affected by stomach, intestinal disease or malabsorption.

- The total amount of the infusion is absorbed and available to the tissues.

- Nutrients are forced into cells by means of a high concentration gradient.

- Higher doses of nutrients can be given than are possible by mouth without intestinal irritation.

Proposed Treatment

Prior to your treatment you will have a consultation with the treating doctor and nutritional recommendations will be discussed. We will not diagnose, treat or cure any specific disease, and the nutritional recommendations we make do not constitute treatment for any disease or affliction.

The purpose of your treatment will be:

- To improve your overall nutritional status;
- To improve your general sense of well-being;
- As a prevention of the ageing process;
- To improve your metabolism;
- For possible remission or reduction of pain where present.

Limitations

An initial series of treatments will be recommended, and these treatments may extend over a number of weeks or months. The benefits of intravenous nutrient therapy are much greater if you follow a healthy lifestyle (non-smoking, weight control, proper exercise, proper diet and nutritional supplementation). As with any other medical procedure, you may not receive any benefit because they do not occur predictably with every patient and in a small percentage of patients, benefits may not occur at all.

About the Author

Dr Harry Singh, BChD, MFGDP

1996 - Qualified as a General Dental Surgeon from Leeds University

1997 - Passed MFGDP(UK)

2000 - Joint owner of "Ninety-Seven" dental clinic

2002 - Undertook basic botulinum and dermal fillers training and started offering facial aesthetics

2002 - Owner of Vogue Dental Clinic

2003-2006 - Vocational Trainer for newly qualified graduates

2007 - Trained in Advanced Skin Health Restoration including medical peels

2007 - Opened 'aesthetics' clinic

2008 – 'aesthetics' clinic won Best Marketing at the Private Dentistry Awards

2008 - 'aesthetics' clinic won Best Team at Dentistry Awards

2009 - Finalist for Best Community Project at Private Dentistry Awards

2010 - Appointed to the editorial board of Premium Practice Dentistry magazine

2010 - Further advanced clinical masterclass training in Botox and Dermal Fillers

2011 – Wrote numerous articles on facial aesthetics in professional magazines

2011 – Invited to film for Vakmentor E-learning platform and DVDs for Dr Seema Sharma

2011-2013 - Advanced clinical training in advanced facial aesthetics and skin health restoration

2012 - Speaker at the Dentistry Show at NEC on the business of setting up a facial aesthetics clinic

2012 – Invited to the board of The Society of Aesthetics Practitioners (TSoAP) council

2012 - Speaker at the Odonti Dental Conference on marketing facial aesthetics

2012 - A finalist in top three for best aesthetics clinic in My Face My Body awards from over 600 entries

2012 – 'aesthetics' clinic voted in top three best facial aesthetics clinics in Private Dentistry Awards

2012 – Voted in top 25 aesthetic dentists in UK 2012-2013

2013 – Speaker at FACE conference on Referral Marketing Tips with your facial aesthetics business

2013 – aesthetics shortlisted as a finalist for best facial aesthetics clinic in Private Dentistry Awards

2013 – Gave up dentistry to solely concentrate on facial aesthetics

2014 – Set up the BTC

2015 – Spoke at Dentistry 15, CCR Expo

2016 – Board member of Aesthetic Medicine

2016 – Spoke at BDA Conference, Dentistry Show, Aesthetic Medicine

2016 – BTC – Highly commended (runner up) for Best Customer Service Provider and Best After Sales Support – FMC Industry awards

2016 – IADFE fellowship

2017 – LMT Galderma

2017 – BTC – Highly commended (runner up) for Best Customer Service Provider

2018 - BTC - Winner - Most Outstanding Business of the Year

2019 – Approved Trainer for the Level 7 qualification in Injectables Training for Aesthetic Medicine

www.aesthetics-dentistry.com

References

1 Darwin, Charles 'The Expression of Emotion in Man and Animals'

2 Finzi, Eric 'The Face of Emotion', 2013

3 Darwin, Charles 'The Expression of Emotion in Man and Animals'

4 Uwe Wollina, Perioral rejuvenation: restoration of attractiveness in ageing females by minimally invasive procedures. Clin Interv Aging, (2013)

5 Verner I. Lip Augmentation. Body Language 2015

6 Raif J. Radianski & Karl H Wesker, The Face: Pictorial Atlas of Clinical Anatomy (Berlin, Quintessence Publishing Co, Ltd 2012) 38

Printed in Poland
by Amazon Fulfillment
Poland Sp. z o.o., Wrocław

94807702R00083